"Simple, concise, and spot-on in its ability to educate. *MedStrong* helps us pause, take account of how we feel, and begin the shift to asking good questions and taking control of our own health......Whether you are a health care provider, someone caring for a loved one, or simply reading for your own personal interest, this book is a must read."

ROBERTA BRIEN
Executive Vice President
Worcester Business Development Corporation

"*MedStrong* has been a game changer for my father. Because of this book, his med list went down from 16 to 12, with the supervision of his doctor. My father feels great!"

DEBBIE LYN TOOMEY, MSN, RN
Injury Prevention Coordinator-Division of Trauma and Acute Care Surgery
Author of *The Happiness Result*

"...Dr. Bartlett's *Medstrong Medication Optimization Plan*—step-by-step—gives patients and caregivers the tools to advocate for themselves and work alongside their providers to reduce medication burden. I love how this book not only educates the reader about risk of overmedication and polypharmacy but also empowers them to take the next steps in their health journey. This book is a must for those caring for older adults."

MELODY L. HARTZLER, PharmD, BCACP, BC-ADM
CEO PharmToTable, LLC

"Dr. Bartlett, has taken a very common health challenge and authored a resource that can be used by healthcare professionals to stop OVER-MEDICATING AMERICA! This practical resource should be required reading in medical and pharmacy schools."

JERRICA DODD, PharmD, MS
Founder/CEO Your Pharmacy Advocate
Executive Editor, PharmaSis Magazine

MedStrong

Shed Your Meds for a Better, Healthier You

Aging Well through Deprescribing

Featuring a 5-Step Medication Optimization Plan

DONNA BARTLETT, PharmD, BCGP

Publisher's Cataloging-in-Publication Data
Bartlett, Donna
MedStrong Shed your meds for a better, healthier you/ Donna Bartlett
Paperback original edition. WELLhood Publishing. Paxton, MA.
Includes index.
LCCN 2022903313 ISBN 978-1-7377563-0-9 ISBN 978-1-7377563-1-6 (ebook)
HEALTH / Medicine
Classification: LCC: RM300-666 DDC: 615.4

ISBN 978-1-7377563-0-9 (paperback)
ISBN 978-1-7377563-1-6 (ebook)

Editor: Tammy Ditmore, eDitmore Editorial Services
Design: Chris Molé, Book Savvy Studio

ATTN: QUANTITY DISCOUNTS ARE AVAILABLE TO YOUR COMPANY, EDUCATIONAL INSTITUTION, OR HEALTH ORGANIZATION for reselling, educational purposes, subscription incentives, gifts, or fundraising campaigns.

For more information please contact the publisher at
WELLhood Publishing,
11 Brooks Road, Paxton, Massachusetts 01612
508-450-0269
Email: info@wellhoodpublishing.com

Dedication

*To all the women and men who find themselves as
caregivers navigating the maze of health care and medications.
— Let's change the narrative and be **MedStrong**!*

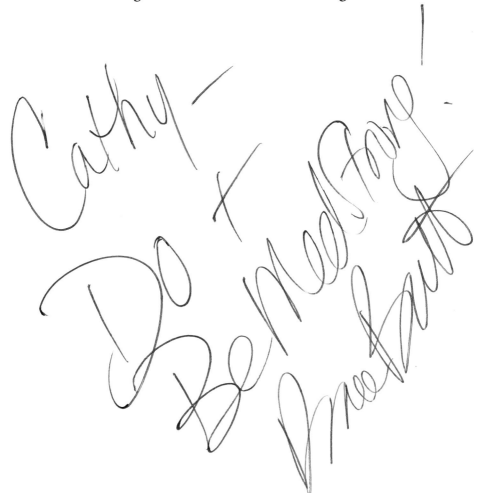

Acknowledgements

WHEN READING ACKNOWLEDGEMENTS OF OTHER BOOKS, it has always amazed me how many people are actually involved in bringing a book into being! Having undertaken this venture of authoring a book, I now have a firsthand appreciation for what a collaborative process it is to find and meet and work hand-in-hand with a team of such talented and invested people. I am so thankful for all of the professionals and supportive people that have provided their expertise, talents, time, interest, and enthusiasm as they helped me to bring this book to fruition. Everyone involved is deserving of praise as well as my sincere gratitude.

Peter Bowerman—I would not have guessed that from a brief 15 minute introductory conversation with Peter, an accomplished commercial free-lance writer, that it would lead to the eventual development of this book title, the back cover copy, and the chapter headings. Peter provided consistent advice and mentoring and is certainly the go-to guy for everything commercial writing!

Tammy Ditmore—a superb editor, was so instrumental in helping to manage the text and flow of the information. She was, like a composer with notes, astute in rearranging words and sections to define the movement of the information in a smooth and coherent way. She navigated the process calmly and expertly, especially when I felt overwhelmed or "stuck", and maintained my voice and goals throughout the book. She guided the process in a way that helped me to concentrate on the content as she managed the details of editing.

Chris Molé—creative genius is not saying enough! Chris' design expertise and vision was so influential in bringing this book to life. From one of our very first conversations, I sensed that she was excited about the "texture" of the book as she spoke about the inclusion of sidebars, process steps, and worksheets. She was insightful and detail-oriented and has helped to create a very visually pleasing cover and layout.

A special thanks to Katharine Dix and Melissa Corcoran, who helped guide me on the initial literary path and who muddled through the very first version with me.

I am also appreciative of the host of beta readers who read through the additional rough draft versions along the way. A special shout-out to Debbie Waldron, who continues to be a great cheerleader as a health-care consumer and caregiver! And to Eugene Lambert, who was a key health-care provider and proponent to view the book and see its worth.

There were many professionals who dedicated their time to review and provide insight with respect to particularly important points and helped to bring clarity to the overall message. I am so thankful for all of their input and advice. A special thank you to Dr. Stephanie Sibicky and Dr. Veronica Riera-Gilley for their positive insight and valuable feedback.

ASCP elite team, Christine Polite and Dr. Chad Worz, are also very much appreciated for their advocacy in supporting and promoting the impact of bringing a book of deprescribing directly to health-care consumers and caregivers through an international senior care pharmacist organization. I so appreciate their excitement and encouragement throughout the process.

A special personal thank you to all of those who make my everyday life wonderful.

First and foremost, my dear family! My husband, John, who is the ultimate supporter and my rock every step of the way. He patiently listened to me in my moments of doubt and gently lifted me back up! To my beautiful children, Lianna and Chad, of whom I am so proud; AND who tell me that they are proud of me too! Thank you for all of your encouragement, strength, fist-pumps, and "Oh-Yah-You-Ares !!!"

And to so many family and friends—near and far—who have supported me in so many ways throughout my life, including this "chapter." (Yes, pun intended!!) Thank you to my parents, siblings, and extended family, my dear Paxton friends, my prayer group, and all those who have supported me in my roles as mother, caregiver, pharmacist, and now author! You each hold a special place in my heart filled with love and gratitude.

To the many colleagues who have been an amazing system of assistance and encouragement throughout this project. A special shout-out to everyone at the Massachusetts College of Pharmacy and Health Sciences University-Worcester/Manchester, who encouraged me and afforded me the time to write and publish! And a special thank you to Dr. Paul Belliveau, the colleague and administrator with whom I first shared the idea of this book. His optimism, interest, and support helped to motivate me as I contemplated beginning this venture and saw it through to its completion.

Table of Contents

TABLES

FIGURES

Foreword

Since the beginning of time, humans have sought relief from ailment in plants, herbs, and chemicals. The earliest forms of medicine extracted from plants was morphine, for pain.

As a pharmacist and because my main focus is deprescribing, I am a self-proclaimed "antipharmacist" where I approach every problem believing a medication is a cause, working to limit medication use whenever possible. Using this philosophy throughout my pharmacy career, I established Medication Managers, LLC, a consulting practice that serves nursing facilities and long-term care pharmacy clients across the country, and later became the executive director and chief executive officer of the American Society of Consultant Pharmacist (ASCP) and the ASCP Foundation. At ASCP, we use a patient-focused approach, driven by deprescribing. We strive to make sure individuals are on the least amount of needed medications, and for most that means eliminating unneeded medication.

While a remedy for every ailment has evolved just as modern health care, a clear understanding of the body, how it ages, and the impact of medicine and chemicals on its function has lagged behind. Sometimes we don't want to know that medications that work may not be good for us—people don't want to admit that French fries and wine can be bad either—as we seek short term relief, often at the expense of long-term complications.

Medication–use is no different. I know from my parents, the motivations behind the use of medication can often times be risky. Ignoring risks that don't manifest immediately with the relief medication provides.

One tried and true solution has always been the sound and steady advice from the pharmacist.

Pharmacists spend at least 6 years in college focused almost exclusively on how medications work in the human body. They pour over the benefits and risks not only in diseases and conditions, but when used in combination with other medications. They enter the health care workforce uniquely skilled at managing medications.

Many readers may not recognize that pharmacists in hospitals, clinics and in long-term care settings often dose highly complex antibiotics, pain regimens, and diabetes protocols. Pharmacists serve as a line of defense between the prescribing practitioner and the ingestion of the drug by the patient. Today's pharmacists work in doctors' offices, clinics, and some do home visits, all in an effort to ensure that medications are providing the benefits we seek without the risks we fear.

I view my profession, especially those pharmacists focusing on older adults, as in the perfect position to impact the aging population. Baby-boomers are now turning 70, and with that seniority comes an increased need for medication management. Our country's health and financial stability depend on us finding innovative ways to use pharmacists to improve quality of life and lower the burden of medications and medication use.

As caregivers, many of us recognize that help is needed. Compliance and daily household situations can create risk. Forgetting to take your medicine, forgetting you took your medication and taking another accidentally, taking more because your symptoms are bad, taking less because you don't like how it makes you feel, storing your medicine in places where it can break down or overheat. The list of problems that one can encounter with medication outside the body can sometimes be as long as the risks inside the body.

Dr. Bartlett is a geriatric pharmacist specialist. She has years of experience working with complex individuals and their equally complex medications. She has multiple stories and insights in this book that can lead you down the road toward sound advice and help you help yourself or one of your loved ones battle the emerging polypharmacy epidemic.

Help is all around us in the form of qualified pharmacists, the trick is understanding that it is always important to ask questions. Herein lies some answers to what's going on, when to ask for help, who to ask and what you can do to help manage medications in an ever-changing medication landscape.

The ASCP Foundation proudly endorses Dr. Bartlett's work in better communicating helpful advice to those struggling with their own or their loved one's medications. This endorsement highlights the great opportunity to communicate the important contributions of senior care pharmacists. Our members are doing fantastic things; we need to tell their stories and continue to support their endeavors. Pharmacy is a family, and ASCP serves as the place for senior care pharmacists to network, share, and improve their practice approaches and to educate those challenged by and navigating the healthcare system.

The mission of the ASCP Foundation is to carry out the charitable – including scientific, literary, and educational – purposes of ASCP, a non-profit organization that strives to empower pharmacist and transform aging.

Pharmacists who specialize in helping people navigate medication related issues can be found at www.helpwithmymeds.org.

My goal is parallel to Dr. Bartlett's, to improve medication management for older adults by bringing the skills of senior care pharmacists to those who need them. The golden age of pharmacy is straight ahead of us; there are just so many older adults who need our expertise!

CHAD WORZ, PharmD, BCGP, FASCP
Executive Director and Chief Executive Officer
American Society of Consultant Pharmacists (ASCP)
ASCP Foundation
Empowering pharmacists
Transforming Aging

Introduction

Have you ever wondered if you're taking too many medications and for too long? Do you ever stop to ask if they are all still necessary? Or to consider whether stopping a medication, even one you have taken for years, might make you feel better?

Medications help keep us healthy and strong and can prevent or reduce the progression of chronic conditions, but they need upkeep too. Medications that have protected us, supported us, and served us well over time may need to be replaced with safer products, removed from our regimen, or reduced to lesser doses.

Being the daughter of a carpenter, I learned firsthand about the importance of building structures to last and fixing things without compromising structural soundness. But even the best-built structures need upkeep—roofs replaced, plumbing repaired, electrical panels updated. Although these elements may have served the structure well for years, changes and updates eventually become necessary for structural integrity. As a pharmacist, I take the same approach to building and updating a medication regimen, especially as my patients age.

Think of an older adult whose health you care about—a parent, grandparent, friend, partner—or maybe yourself. Do they take medications? How many? Five or more? How long have they been taking these medications? When was the last time they took something that was not prescribed, an over-the-counter remedy or supplement? Possibly every day? I have heard some patients say they take so much medication every day that they "sound like a vial of pills!"

Now think about that person's overall health. Have they been hospitalized recently? Fallen? Do they have concerns of feeling old or express issues like forgetfulness, confusion, insomnia, or weakness?

Polypharmacy, the taking of five or more prescription or nonprescription medications on a regular basis,[1] can lead to many of these conditions. It's not just the number of medications that can be harmful, but the number of unnecessary medications. Our health system is very good at prescribing medications to treat health conditions, but it's not always good at deprescribing medications that may no longer be necessary.

What is deprescribing? Deprescribing is the thoughtful process of reducing, switching, or stopping a medication that may no longer be needed or may no longer be the best treatment option. The deprescribing process should be overseen by a health-care provider in communication with the patient or a caregiver.[2] Not all medications can or should be stopped, but you may be taking medications that are no longer necessary or pose more of a risk than a benefit as you age.

Aging Changes Everything

Why is deprescribing important? Throughout the aging process, your body changes. Think of how much your body changes in your first 20, 30, or 40 years of life. Now consider how many changes a 65-year-old will experience if they live to be 85, 95, even 105. That's why considering whether a medication is still appropriate, needed, or dosed properly is an important key to healthy aging. A medication you may have started taking at 40 may not serve you well by the time you reach 80.

Your body's ability to absorb, distribute, metabolize, and eliminate medications changes throughout your lifetime, and those changes are especially acute in your older years. Changes in gut motility and acid production can change how medications are absorbed. Increased body fat and decreased hydration in older adults changes the distribution or delivery of medications throughout the body. Liver size and function decrease with age, which can reduce how well the body metabolizes medications. Age-related reduction of kidney size and function affects how well medications are eliminated from the body. Side effects may appear even after a person has taken a medication for years. Instead of taking another pill to combat the side effect, it may be possible to change, reduce, or eliminate the medication causing the ill effect.

Polypharmacy and certain medications can also lead to falls, which can be especially devastating to older adults. Though many factors contribute to falls, including health conditions, health status, sensory impairment, and environment, falls are not a "normal" part of the aging process. Deprescribing certain medications may help prevent a fall from occurring.

Do You Have Questions? You Should!

With so many factors to consider, where do you begin? How can you initiate productive conversations with health-care providers regarding the care for yourself or others? People frequently tell me, "At the pharmacy, I am asked, 'Do you have any questions?' Quite honestly, I don't know what to ask."

I understand! When my daughter was diagnosed with a brain tumor and we were waiting for more detailed tests, the medical team asked if we had any questions. My honest answer was, "Millions!" But, honestly, I could not formulate even one question at that time. Fortunately, we had the time to make a list of questions, which helped us and her medical team devise a patient-specific plan for a successful outcome.

As you read through this book, make time to develop your questions. Don't wait for a problem such as a side effect or a fall to occur. Some medications are considered potentially inappropriate or risky for older adults, so you can always start a conversation by asking a provider if you or someone you care for is taking any potentially inappropriate medications. In chapter 5, I will list and explain other questions you can ask.

Deprescribing is a way to optimize your medications. Stopping, reducing, or changing a medication may not have immediate results. However, over time, deprescribing may help you feel better, be more active, and maintain a better quality of life. After following a deprescribing process, some people think more clearly, have better balance, and no longer suffer from dizziness. Others feel less fatigued, stronger, and able to accomplish more every day. Others just feel better in general.

Deprescribing is different for everyone, so it is difficult to generalize how it should be done or what effects it might have. The process needs to be individualized based on a person's needs, health status or function, and health conditions.[3]

Polypharmacy is a global problem. Researchers from all over the world examine polypharmacy issues and the need to reduce prescriptions. Globally, as the number of older adults increases, experts expect the number of medications, the number of chronic diseases per individual, and problems related to polypharmacy will also rise. Building awareness of polypharmacy and taking advantage of the benefits of deprescribing can potentially reduce frailty, falls, hospitalizations, and adverse drug events. Deprescribing is a medical solution to the "condition" of polypharmacy.

You may be asking why a pharmacist or associate professor of pharmacy would write a book about reducing medications. The answer is that I want to see older adults enjoying life instead of suffering needless side effects from their medications. As a certified geriatric pharmacist, I have seen brown bags and pill boxes filled to the brim with unnecessary medications and have counseled many individuals, groups, and caregivers about medicines that need to be used with caution and prescriptions that may be more appropriate for older adults. If deprescribing can help someone feel better, move about more easily, enjoy a conversation, take a walk, or smile again, I am delighted to be part of the solution.

I do not want people to wait for the fall, the confusion, or the accident to make a change. Instead, I want to empower them to ask the right questions about their medication use so they can determine whether their medications are needed or could be changed or reduced.

What Does This Book Provide?

This book provides information, examples, and questions to help you review your medications with your health-care providers and work with them to create action plans for safe, thoughtful deprescribing. In the following chapters, you will learn how any medication has the potential of becoming more of a risk than a benefit over time and how the effects of medications can vary depending upon a person's health status, chronic and acute health conditions, and other medications.

And you will learn the five steps of the MedStrong Medication Optimization Plan (MOP) to identify and manage medications that may no longer be necessary or beneficial, especially the ones that may increase the risk of an adverse event and lead to poorer health outcomes. You can use the MedStrong MOP for yourself or for anyone in your care. It will help you keep a check on your medications, take only what you need, and remain healthy and strong as you age.

A NOTE TO HEALTH-CARE PROVIDERS

Though this book is aimed at health-care consumers, providers can learn from it too. Chapters 9 and 10 are particularly geared toward providers. However, both providers and consumers will learn about the need and purpose of deprescribing throughout the book.

There is an urgent call to change the medication culture and for deprescribing to happen regularly. Our daily health-care practices require updating to consistently identify high-risk patients and to treat preventatively. Identifying potentially inappropriate medications in a proactive manner so that we can reduce adverse events and hospitalizations related to unnecessary medications adds value to the quality of health care and can increase a patient's quality of life.

Treatment guidelines, age sensitivity and discrimination, clinical inertia, and misidentifying side effects of medications as new disease states all contribute to polypharmacy. To begin the deprescribing process, start with a step-by-step approach that includes a review of a current, accurate medication list; the patient's goals, life expectancy, current health conditions, and patient assessment; and an evaluation of any potentially inappropriate medications. A deprescribing plan can then be developed safely through shared decision-making.

Many of the treatment guidelines used in healthcare are not necessarily intended for older adults, so providers should carefully consider whether the treat-to-target goals of a guideline are appropriate for older patients and whether following such guidance could raise risks of potential harm. Scott and colleagues[4] provide an analysis of numerous studies supporting deprescribing, including reduction of medications by up to 58%, with over 80% of patients successfully deprescribed without having to restart medications and almost 90% reporting health improvement. Medications that were deprescribed in these studies varied, as did the patients' living arrangements, which ranged from community dwelling to long-term care.

Something to consider: Several studies show deprescribing can lead to healthy outcomes. "No change" may also be a positive outcome.

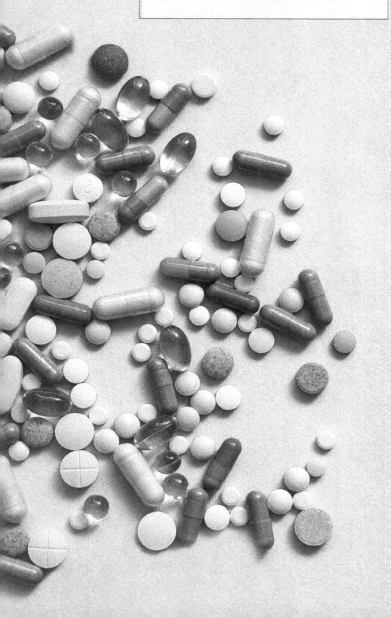

PART I
Overmedicated

CHAPTER 1

Mind Your Meds

IF YOU ARE NOT FEELING WELL, you want something to make you feel better. At various points in your life, you have probably been prescribed multiple medications that proved beneficial, perhaps even lifesaving, and allowed for a better quality of life by enabling you to work, play, or travel. Maybe your medication gave you the health you needed to serve as a mentor, parent, teacher, CEO, mechanic, religious leader, state trooper, the very person you are today. But as you grow older, a retooling of your medications may be required so you can continue your activities or take on new ones. Reexamining your medications can help you continue to receive benefits while minimizing the risks of potential adverse drug events.

There are countless needs for properly dosed medications. For example, medications help reduce blood pressure to prevent heart attacks and strokes and reduce disease symptoms and progression of chronic conditions such as colitis, rheumatoid arthritis, HIV, and many others. Medicines replace deficiencies, such as levothyroxine to treat an underactive thyroid; levodopa is converted to dopamine to treat Parkinson's disease. Some people who try to avoid prescription drugs by engaging in nonmedication therapy and lifestyle changes may find they are still unable to successfully reach their ideal blood pressure or cholesterol levels or to overcome depression or anxiety without medication. Prescription drugs are truly helpful and allow us to live productive lives.

Our current health-care culture is linked to prescribing treatments. Many patients expect to be prescribed something to feel better, and prescribers want to make their patients feel better with medicine. Furthermore, it is generally easier, and often quicker, to take a medicine than to change habits or lifestyle. But it can be tricky for patients and providers alike to realize when a medication that has been beneficial for years begins to cause more harm than good. It's not always easy to see when a long-used medication may need to be stopped, reduced, or changed.

And patients and providers are not the only ones involved in the medication culture. Pharmaceutical manufacturers provide a wealth of information regarding starting a medication, the dosage needed, when you may be able to increase the dose, and the maximum dose criteria. However, few manufacturers provide such detailed information about how or when to stop medications.

Furthermore, disease guidelines, which are widely used by healthcare providers, offer information on how to treat a health condition and the progression of the condition but do not necessarily offer advice about when treatment is no longer necessary or how to stop treatment. Yes, that's right, there are few guidelines to advise when you might stop, reduce, or change a medication that you have been taking for a chronic condition for years.

Think back to a time when you started taking medication that helped reduce the negative effects of either an acute or a chronic need. Do you remember that feeling of "Wow! I didn't realize how bad I was feeling." When I was pregnant with my first child, I was nauseous for the first trimester, but I tried to minimize it by thinking, "This is not as bad as some of the women I know who have been hospitalized during pregnancy for dehydration from severe morning sickness." But after the nausea finally lifted around the fourth month, I remember thinking, "I guess I really wasn't feeling very well." During a different pregnancy, I experienced a daily headache for five months. What a relief when it finally dissipated, and I felt "normal" again.

Why do I tell you these stories? To illustrate how changes in your body can make you feel and how you can "not feel your best" for so long that you almost forget how good you can feel. You may even shrug off your ailment by thinking, "It could be worse."

Continuing medications unnecessarily or inappropriately can make you feel a lot worse than you need to. Stopping, reducing, or switching medications may just make you feel better and give you that "Wow, I didn't realize how bad I was actually feeling" moment. But there is not an automatic or exact process of knowing when a medication is no longer needed, unless it is an antibiotic that you take for a specific number of days, for example.

I have experienced this firsthand. I took a medication that was necessary for years, but eventually the medication caused side effects due to my changing body. I worked with my doctor, and we were able to deprescribe the medicine over time. I am still evaluated regularly but have not needed to restart the medication. That may change, but I prefer not having the side effects and am pleased that I am faring well without the medicine that was once very necessary.

At this point, you may be wondering, "What? Deprescribing is not an automatic thing? Why would any of us be taking medicine that is no longer necessary in the first place? Aren't doctors supposed to keep track of this?"

And if you are not a health-care professional, you may also be wondering, "Where do I start?" How can you raise the issue of appropriateness of medications and advocate for yourself with your health-care providers? This process becomes even more difficult for older people who are experiencing cognitive changes or relying on others to track medications and advocate for their health care.

That's what this book is all about. In these pages, you will learn how to work with your health-care team to reduce unnecessary medications and optimize necessary ones for your best health.

The ultimate goal of this book is to enlighten and empower you as a health-care consumer.

The Challenges of Deprescribing

It is difficult to think that a medication you have been taking for years may now be causing more harm than benefit or just providing you no benefit at all. Unfortunately, there is not an automatic or exact process of knowing when a medication is no longer needed, and because some effects from medications may change subtly over time, you may not even recognize that you are not as well as you could be. Being truthful about how you feel and honest when something does not seem quite right are the keys to initiating the deprescribing conversation that could help you feel better.

Many of my friends, siblings, and older family members have told me that they never realized a medication might not be benefiting them any longer until they read one of my blog posts or heard one of my podcasts on deprescribing. They then tell me they are now reducing or changing a medication after talking with their prescriber.

Some events, such as hospitalizations and rehab care, can be critical times for a medication review and reconciliation. During transitions of care, when you are changing from one set of health-care providers to another, it's easy to become confused and unsure about what changes may have been made to your prescriptions or what steps need to come next. The post-hospitalization follow-up appointment is an ideal time to review the need for all medications—new and old. Can you stop certain medications now that you are no longer in an acute care setting? Are the changes made while you were in the hospital appropriate? Are there any duplications in your prescription regimen? This careful approach allows you to understand any changes, provides a means to document changes, and allows for continued follow-up if necessary.

When someone is in a continuing care or hospice situation, difficult conversations are warranted whenever changes occur to your or your loved one's health or care. Are all current medications still needed? When a patient's life expectancy is short, it may be unnecessary to continue medications meant to prevent long-term health issues or boost longevity. Especially question the need to continue vitamins and medications used for dementia and to address cholesterol levels, to name a few.

Wise and Well

The many articles and studies regarding polypharmacy (typically viewed as five or more medications) consistently point to a correlation with falls, cognitive deficits, and adverse side effects, all of which become a concern for individual and community health. Medications can affect cognitive changes, reaction times, and delayed processing, especially in older adults, and those problems can also lead to traffic accidents, a public health concern. Just as we look at seatbelts as a mechanism to reduce injuries while driving, we can look at deprescribing as the "seatbelt" to reduce the negative effects of polypharmacy.

Everyone—you, your caregivers, pharmacists, prescribers, insurance companies, and the pharmaceutical industry—needs to be educated about and participate in the stopping, reducing, and switching of medications. Medications do a fabulous job of keeping us alive and well so we can reach our older years, but time changes the body, and we need to keep reviewing medications to avoid toxicities and negative effects, such as falls, accidents, and adverse drug events.

Let's begin the journey of being wise, well, and MedStrong. In Part I of this book, we will explore the background of polypharmacy and why you should worry about being overmedicated and overprescribed. In Part II you will learn about deprescribing, how you and your caregivers can start the process with your health-care providers, and how to critically review your medications. In Part III, you will learn the benefits, barriers, and potential pitfalls of this intricate process. Finally, Part IV provides thought-provoking steps forward for health-care providers and patients who are ready to take action.

By the time you complete this book, you will have the tools to review your medications with your providers, advocate for yourself or someone you care for, and navigate your health-care needs. This process will empower you to become an educated health-care consumer. To continue the analogy from the introduction, the deprescribing process will help you "fix and update your house" so you can enjoy a strong and sound body as you age.

CHAPTER 2

In Over Our Meds

HAVE COUNSELED OLDER ADULTS about medications for years and have seen many people on multiple medications—with some people taking nine, twelve, or even more. Medications are sometimes added by a prescriber to counter a side effect of another medication, creating a "prescribing cascade" that might have been avoided by simply changing the initial, offending medication. Patients may also "self-prescribe" an over-the-counter (OTC) medication for what they think is an ailment but may actually be a side effect of a prescription.

In addition, one patient may be taking multiple medications prescribed by multiple providers, including primary care physicians, specialists, dentists, optometrists, nurse practitioners, physician assistants, medical residents—and in some cases—pharmacists. Think of all the health-care providers you see. Do you receive a prescription from each practice? Most of them?

Has a commercial or advertisement ever convinced you or a loved one to "act now" and order a medication or OTC product? Older adults may be especially likely to follow recommendations from friends or family regarding OTC medications, supplements, and herbals without checking to see if the products duplicate or interact with their prescription medications. Compounding the problem is the easy availability of these products at the pharmacy, grocery store, gas station, convenience store, health-food store, and online sources.

Gone are the days when most people frequented only one pharmacy and "got to know" the pharmacist. Mail-order, specialty pharmacies, local pharmacies, and clinic pharmacies have gained in popularity due to insurance coverage, convenience, reduce-priced generics, and specific medications for specific health conditions.

When multiple pharmacies are involved, then the system check for potential drug interactions may be incomplete, especially if insurance is not being used for all prescriptions.

So many variables can add to a person's list of medications, and these same variables can also lead to confusion because of multiple medications. Polypharmacy happens—and there may be no one to blame. The important part is recognizing it might be a problem and doing something about it.

What Is Polypharmacy?

Polypharmacy is not necessarily defined by a particular number of medications, although the use of five or more is often used as a benchmark. But more significant than the number of medications is whether the medications being taken continue to be necessary and appropriate.[4]

Polypharmacy can be appropriate, as when someone takes several medications that are all needed, well-managed, and helpful in treating multiple chronic health conditions—for example, high blood pressure, diabetes, and asthma. Each of these conditions typically warrants multiple medications, resulting in a high number of medications prescribed.

Why Worry about Polypharmacy?

So, if polypharmacy can be appropriate and many people thrive while taking multiple medications, why should we worry about it? We need to pay attention because research has shown that polypharmacy can lead to other well-documented problems, including

- prescribing cascades;
- overuse, underuse, or misuse of medications;
- complex regimens with questionable benefits;
- increased risk of frailty and hospital admissions;
- greater experiences of geriatric syndromes; and
- higher risks of adverse drug events, including drug interactions.

Let's take a closer look at some of these potential problems.

Polypharmacy can lead to prescribing cascades

A prescribing cascade is where one medication can lead to another. Because more side effects can occur when a patient takes more medications, even more medications may be prescribed to treat these adverse effects. The opposite is also true: a prescribing cascade can lead to polypharmacy when "unnecessary" medications are added to treat a side effect instead of changing the original medication to avoid the side effect.

As you can see, it is easy to wind up in a polypharmacy situation. To avoid prescribing cascades, be sure you know exactly why you take each of your medications and why your provider thinks each is necessary for you. Becoming an educated health consumer can help you keep your medications in check.

IN REAL LIFE

The following scenario illustrates how prescribing cascades may sometimes be necessary initially but continued needlessly—and possibly to a harmful effect.

Diuretics (sometimes called "water pills") have for many years been a first-line medication against high blood pressure. But some prescribed diuretics can reduce potassium, so health-care providers subsequently add a prescription for supplemental potassium. This diuretic-plus-potassium combination is considered a prescribing cascade because the diuretic lowers potassium levels, causing the patient to take another medication to counteract or correct the effect of the original medication. The combination can be very effective if managed well but can become problematic if it is not.

Mr. K, an older gentleman, had taken the diuretic, hydrochlorothiazide (HCTZ), for approximately 25 years to reduce blood pressure. He was also taking potassium chloride to keep his potassium levels normal and was prescribed other medication as he grew older. When Mr. K lost weight and began experiencing orthostatic hypotension, or low blood pressure, when he stood up, it was decided that the diuretic was no longer necessary because his blood pressure was within normal range. Deprescribing HCTZ would potentially reduce the risk of orthostatic hypotension.

But when it came time for his next 90-day refills, Mr. K called in for a refill of his potassium tablets. The pharmacist asked if he still needed the HCTZ but was told that medication had been stopped by the doctor. Recognizing that the potassium tablets were probably no longer necessary if the HCTZ had been stopped, the pharmacist checked with the physician, who confirmed that the HCTZ was indeed deprescribed and then stated, "Oh yeah, the potassium can also be discontinued."

Had the potassium not been stopped, Mr. K's potassium levels would have increased over time and a potential abnormal heart rhythm could have occurred, resulting in hospitalization.

Polypharmacy can cause overuse, underuse, or misuse of medications and can result in complex regimens with questionable benefits[5]

Overuse can occur when someone is confused or forgetful, which can lead them to forget they have taken a medication and then take it again. My mother would help my grandfather manage his medications by placing his medicines in a pill organizer. Later in the week, she would discover that medications were missing from many days in addition to the ones that were supposed to be taken.

Underuse can follow the same scenario. Perhaps you can't remember if you've taken a particular prescription today, so you just decide not to take it. Maybe you just forget about one of your medications. This can happen especially with medicines that are supposed to be taken multiple times per day.

Misuse of medication can happen because of confusion about the correct dose or the timing of the medication. Or you might misunderstand specific instructions or confuse one medication for another. I once counseled an older adult about her intake of daily aspirin. Her doctor told her to "take baby aspirin every day," so the woman went to the pharmacy, bought baby aspirin, and took four baby aspirin, four times daily, as instructed on the box. However, those instructions are for pain and fever relief. When I reviewed her medication, I explained that her doctor wanted her to take aspirin for heart protection, so probably wanted her to take only one tablet, once a day. I asked if she had any bruising, if her gums bled easily when she brushed or flossed, or if she had nose bleeds. She had not experienced any of those side effects but was very embarrassed by her misuse of the aspirin. I explained that she had done what she was told, which was to "take aspirin daily." Because she was not given specific instructions, she followed the directions on the box, leading to misuse of a medication that could have led to harmful effects.

Complex regimens can occur from complicated medication directions that make it hard for some users to understand or follow all the directions. For example, some medications need to be taken regularly—sometimes multiple times a day—while other medications are used only for flare-ups of the same condition. Individuals need to know when to take certain medications and not confuse a rescue medication with a maintenance medication. The more prescriptions a user has, the easier it is to get confused about the necessary regimen.

Questions about the *benefits* of multiple medications also grow as more medications are added, because more medications can lead to more side effects and more adverse events. More medications also increase the risk of additive effects and interactions.

Polypharmacy increases the risk of adverse events, including drug interactions

Drug interactions can be drug–drug, drug–disease, drug–food, or drug–alcohol interactions.

Drug–drug interactions occur when a combination of drugs causes one or more of the meds to work differently in a person's body. There may be an increased effect, a decreased effect, or an additive effect.

Increased effects typically occur when one medication causes another medication to have a higher exposure to the receptors in the body, which may lead to more side effects or toxicities. For example, amlodipine, a common blood pressure medication, can cause simvastatin, a common cholesterol-lowering medication, to have more exposure or availability, which could cause users to experience muscle aches and pains from the higher amounts of simvastatin available in the body.

Decreased effects occur when combining medications causes one or more of the drugs to be less effective. Tamoxifen is a medication used for breast cancer patients to reduce the risk of the cancer returning. If the antidepressant fluoxetine, for example, is also taken, then the tamoxifen is less likely to be effective because fluoxetine interferes with its activity. This interaction could result in tamoxifen being ineffective and potentially result in a return of the breast cancer.

An additive type of drug interaction happens when multiple medications are combined and produce similar outcomes or side effects. For example, more than one drug may be used to reduce blood pressure, or several antibiotics may be combined to treat a complicated infection. These combination therapies are not necessarily harmful and, in fact, may have a beneficial effect. When multiple medications have similar side effects, however, such as drowsiness or dizziness, the combination of drugs can cause an additive effect that could be harmful.

Drug–disease interactions occur when a medication being used to treat one condition makes another condition worse. For example, many OTC medication labels state, "Do not take if" or "Consult your doctor or pharmacist if" you have certain conditions. For example, a decongestant for cold or allergy could increase blood pressure, worsening existing hypertension. Pain relief medications, such as ibuprofen or naproxen, may worsen types of heart disease, including heart failure. It is important to heed the warnings on OTC labels so you do not worsen other conditions while self-treating for a different problem. It is just as important to read the prescription information sheets you receive from the pharmacy to be certain that your prescribed medications will not worsen other conditions.

Drug–food interactions are typically noted on prescription drugs with auxiliary label cautions—the used-to-be colorful stickers and now yellow precaution stickers—that may be added to your prescription label. Prescriptions with labels warning about the intake of dairy or grapefruit are common. Many prescriptions instruct users to allow for a two-hour window of separation between dairy consumption and drug intake. That's because dairy products contain calcium, which can reduce the absorption of certain medications, causing a reduced benefit.

Warnings about eating grapefruit are typically placed on cholesterol-lowering agents known as statins. When combined with grapefruit, many statins are not metabolized properly and can accumulate in the body, causing a "stacking," dose by dose, to high levels that may cause side effects, especially muscle pain and weakness. (Note: Not all statins are affected by grapefruit; for example, grapefruit can be enjoyed without worry when one is taking rosuvastatin or pravastatin. If you love grapefruit, asking your health-care provider something as simple as, "Can I eat grapefruit with this?" can allow for a better match between you and your prescription.)

Alcohol affects all systems of the body; therefore, it is no surprise that several medications—prescription and OTC—can cause ***drug–alcohol interactions***. On its own, alcohol can cause confusion, upset stomach, stomach bleeds, seizures, blurred vision, increased heart rate, low heart rate, arrhythmias, dry mouth, unsteadiness, stumbling, falls, insomnia, sleepiness, and more. As with medications, alcohol is less easily tolerated, causes more side effects, and is more difficult to metabolize and eliminate as we age. Many medications cause side effects similar to those caused by alcohol, so taking any of those medications with alcohol can lead to additive effects and more severe reactions. The National Institutes of Health offer a booklet online that provides drug–alcohol interaction information.[6]

Polypharmacy and unnecessary medications may lead to geriatric syndromes

We like to blame many ailments on advancing age, including constipation, cognition deficits, falls, hospitalizations, uncontrolled bladder, weight loss, dizziness, blood pressure changes, unsteadiness, arrhythmias, mood changes, and other issues that negatively affect quality of life. But many of these "age-related" conditions may actually be caused or worsened by polypharmacy or unnecessary medications. Many medications are directly associated with these conditions, which may resolve if a medication is reduced, changed, or stopped. Table 2.1 lists some types of medications that may contribute to age-related conditions or geriatric syndromes.[7]

Table 2.1

Medications that May Contribute to Age-related Conditions

Geriatric Syndrome	Types of Medications
Delirium, dementia, cognitive deficit, confusion	Medications for overactive bladder Antidepressants Medications for allergies Antipsychotics Medications for stomach spasms Muscle relaxants Benzodiazepines and medications used for anxiety and insomnia Corticosteroids
Falls	Medications used for seizures Medications to control high blood pressure Antipsychotics Medications used for insomnia Benzodiazepines and medications used for anxiety and insomnia, including TCAs (e.g., amitriptyline) and SSRIs (e.g., paroxetine)
Overactive bladder	Medications used for Alzheimer's Diuretics ("water pills")
Dizziness and drop in blood pressure	Medications for overactive bladder Medications for high blood pressure Medications for diabetes such as glyburide and glipizide Antidepressants Medications for allergies Antipsychotics Opioids for pain relief Medications for insomnia
Difficulty swallowing	Medications to strengthen bones NSAIDs (e.g., ibuprofen, naproxen) Potassium
Taste/smell aversion	Blood pressure meds Antibiotics Medications for allergies Eyedrops

Geriatric Syndrome	Types of Medications
Reduced appetite	Antibiotics Medications for seizures Digoxin Benzodiazepines Metformin Opioids Antidepressants
Constipation	Overactive bladder medications Allergy medications Opioids Calcium channel blockers, (e.g., verapamil) Iron

Even though medications may be taken together for many years with few problems, the combination may eventually produce ill effects. Interestingly, a mouse study was conducted by researchers regarding polypharmacy.[8] Older mice given a number of medications commonly taken by older adults, including simvastatin for cholesterol, metoprolol for blood pressure and heart rate, omeprazole for stomach acid, acetaminophen for pain, and citalopram for anxiety or depression, were found to have lower levels of mobility, balance, and strength when compared to older mice not given these medications or younger mice that were given these medications. Further study is needed, but this is an indication that multiple medications may have greater negative effects as we age.

Polypharmacy increases risks of frailty and hospital admissions

Older adults are at risk for adverse drug events, such as falls, and medication toxicities that can lead to hospital admissions. In a frail older adult, some medications may have an increased risk of side effects.

In a study of older adults and polypharmacy, patients were screened for various side effects that may implicate a medication.[9] The study showed side effects common with medications and polypharmacy in older adults including diarrhea, constipation, stomach pains, nausea, dry mouth, dry eyes, dizziness, headache, trouble sleeping, rash, itch, cough, ankle or foot swelling, anxiety, depression, agitation, tremor, confusion, and palpitations. These side effects, which can range from annoying to life threatening, may be reversed if a medication is stopped, reduced, or switched. Blood work, labs, and measurements of vital signs may also reveal issues with medication side effects and toxicities, helping to identify which medication(s) may be overprescribed.

Of note, pharmacists are trained and available to assist with these concerns. Be sure to ask your pharmacist about any of these concerns of polypharmacy, drug interactions, and side effects.

How Does Polypharmacy Occur?

In an article called "Easy to Start, Hard to Stop," which focuses on polypharmacy and deprescribing, Dr. Barbara Farrell shares a common scenario that demonstrates how easily polypharmacy can occur.[10]

> *A medication is started to see how it will help, possibly even as a diagnostic trial, then the medication is continued. Ten years then go by and the primary care doctor retires. The patient sees a new primary care physician who is not quite certain why a patient is on a particular medication but is uneasy about stopping the medication. Now the patient is in their 80s and has been on the medication for 30 years, yet no one really knows why.*

This is a common scenario, where the patient is not having difficulties at the time of the appointment, and all seems well and good.

In addition, older adults may be reluctant to make any changes in their routines, which may be affected by the way they process, understand, and apply information. In an analysis titled "Too Much Medicine in Older People?," the authors cite studies that show how our ability to take in information and make decisions changes through the years.[11] Older adults may find it overwhelming when health-care providers offer several options and identify multiple pros and cons. Instead, older adults tend to focus on positive information, prefer fewer options, and seek less information. Polypharmacy may also contribute to slowed processing and negatively impact decision-making. So, it's easy to see how older adults may choose the path of least resistance and prefer no changes in their medications. And the more medications they take, the higher the likelihood they can be overwhelmed with the idea of making changes.

Working at a pharmacy outreach program opened my eyes to the realities associated with the path of least resistance. During Medicare open enrollment, we would provide the lowest cost option available for a Medicare Part D Plan using the Medicare Plan Finder to identify the charges for the medications an individual was taking. Some of the people I counseled could have saved hundreds or even thousands of dollars by switching plans due to the differences in formularies, copayments, premiums, and deductibles. However, just knowing about these savings did not necessarily entice individuals to change their plans because they found it easier to stay with the plan they already had, especially if their medications remained covered. I was always surprised by this, but I now understand that it is more common to not act in our older years, even if there is a benefit from taking action. I also saw more resistance from people who were on multiple medications, which may mean polypharmacy impacted their reluctance to change plans.

When Is Polypharmacy Appropriate?

Sometimes polypharmacy makes sense, but it needs to be managed well. Some health conditions, such as type 2 diabetes, are commonly treated with multiple medications. Because diabetes also impacts heart health, prescriptions for type 2 diabetes include not only medications to lower blood sugar but also medications for blood pressure and cholesterol. Similarly, after a heart attack, an individual is usually placed on medications for blood pressure, heart rate, cholesterol, and a blood thinner or antithrombotic. Leaving the hospital with five new medications can be daunting, especially for someone who has not been taking prescription drugs, yet it is medically beneficial. Multiple medications are also frequently needed to treat chronic obstructive pulmonary disease (COPD), which requires daily inhalers and rescue inhalers that can be detrimental if taken incorrectly. Heart failure treatments include medications for blood pressure and heart rate, as well as diuretics, which may be increased temporarily to prevent worsening fluid overload. And as individuals age, they may face multiple health conditions and need multiple medications for each condition.

Recognizing the number of medications that may be prescribed for common health problems can show why polypharmacy may be appropriate for some people. However, despite the initial need for multiple medications, there may come a time when the medications are inappropriate for the individual or may be causing unwanted side effects. It is especially important that older adults who see multiple specialists for various health conditions have their medications carefully reviewed by a health-care provider or pharmacist.

Medication reviews and potential deprescribing processes optimize appropriate medication use. Polypharmacy patients should also be informed how lifestyle choices can affect health outcomes and potentially reduce the need for medications. By adopting healthy choices including diet, appropriate fluid and sodium intake, stress reduction, exercise, smoking cessation, and socialization, individuals can and do reduce the number of medications they need, and they often feel better and enjoy a better quality of life with those changes.

Even when individuals face health conditions that commonly warrant polypharmacy, it is important to recognize the following four factors that can change the benefit-versus-harm calculation of certain medications for older adults: pharmacodynamics and pharmacokinetics, multiple comorbidities and frailty, additive adverse effects, and changes in a patient's goals or outlook.[12]

Pharmacodynamics, what the drug does to the body, and pharmacokinetics, what the body does with the drug, can vary and change as we age, which will be explored further in chapter 3. It is important to think about what you put into your body and consider how your body deals with each substance. Good, bad, or indifferent, as your body changes, these factors change too.

Medication may not provide robust benefits for older adults, especially those with multiple comorbidities or those who become frail. Studies of medications tend to include healthy individuals and younger participants, and many dosage guidelines are geared to adults but not necessarily older adults. Understandably, dosing, side effects, and benefits for older adults can vary greatly from those seen with the typical adult dose. The research to show medication effects—good and bad—for older adults is weak or lacking in many cases.

Older adults are more sensitive to side effects, especially those that affect the brain and heart. Additive adverse effects, when multiple medications cause similar side effects, are especially troublesome and potentially harmful.

Also, as people age, there can be changes in the goals of a particular therapy and/or in the goals of the patient. Part II of this book will further explore changing goals. However, it seems clear that a person's health and wellness goals at age 30 are probably markedly different from their goals for health and wellness at age 50 and age 80.

CHAPTER 3

In Pharm's Way

YOUR BODY CHANGES THROUGHOUT YOUR LIFETIME. It's easier to understand this concept when you think about pediatric patients. You would typically not give the same dose of a medication to a one-year-old as you would to an 18-year-old. Although adults' bodies may not outwardly change as drastically as children's bodies, changes in absorption, distribution, metabolism, and elimination (ADME) occur throughout the aging process. Thus, the medication dose you take at age 40 may not be the appropriate dose for you at 70, even if you are still roughly the same height and weight and even though prescribing guidelines are often the same for adults, regardless of age.

ADME

ADME stands for the absorption, distribution, metabolism, and elimination of a medication; in other words, what happens when we take a medication.

- **Absorption** describes how a drug finds its way to our bloodstream and receptors. For oral medications it involves the gut—otherwise known as the gastrointestinal tract.
- **Distribution** describes where the drug goes in the body: the brain, the blood, muscle. Blood flow, water/fluid volume, fat, and proteins all affect the body's distribution of a medication.
- **Metabolism** describes how medication changes in the body. Some changes may activate a medication or prepare it to be eliminated from the body, a process that relies on liver function.
- **Elimination** describes the excretion of the drug from the body, which typically relies on kidney and bowel functions.

How Aging Can Change ADME

Absorption can be affected by gut health and medications, such as proton pump inhibitors that reduce acid levels in the stomach. As you age, your gut functions slow, and medications may not be as readily absorbed. Slower absorption rates may be more problematic for acute or quick-acting medications, such as pain-relievers or antibiotics that need to be absorbed for appropriate therapeutic and beneficial levels.

Slower absorption may not cause as many problems with medications taken for chronic conditions because these types of medications are monitored for a particular outcome. Doses can be raised or lowered, depending upon clinical (how you are feeling) and therapeutic (how your labs and vitals are responding to the medication) outcomes.

Distribution also changes over time. Most people tend to have more body fat later in life, and more fat means medications that are fat-loving—lipophilic—may remain in the body longer before they are eliminated. In addition, aging can lead to decreased thirst perception, lessened fluid intake, and higher likelihood of dehydration. Medications that are water-loving—hydrophilic—tend to accumulate in the body at higher concentrations when there is less hydration and more dehydration. In both cases, more fat or less hydration, lower doses of medications may be needed to prevent increased side effects and toxicity.

Metabolism frequently changes in an aging body due to smaller liver size, less blood flow to the liver, and poor liver function. A slowing metabolism reduces the ability of the body to convert a drug to a product ready for elimination, leading to more side effects and toxicity of the medication. Conversely, some medications need to be metabolized to an active form to be helpful; when this process is reduced, then the effectiveness of the medication is also reduced.

To make things even more challenging, older adults are likely to be taking multiple medications that are competing to be metabolized.

Elimination of medications typically occurs through the kidneys. Like the liver, kidneys also decrease in size, have less blood flow, and may not function as well as people age. If drugs and the byproducts of metabolism are not eliminated, then medication concentrations can increase, causing side effects and toxicity. Kidney function can be calculated for proper dosing and management of medications, and the equation used to determine kidney function includes age as a factor. Age inversely affects kidney function: the higher the age, the lower the kidney function.

A Closer Look: Pharmacokinetics and Pharmacodynamics

ADME (absorption, distribution, metabolism, and elimination) are the components of *pharmacokinetics*: what the body does to the drug, when a medication will begin to work, how long its peak will last, its half-life for elimination purposes, and how the drug is eliminated. These functions or kinetics can be altered with age.

Another factor is *pharmacodynamics*: what the drug does to the body. Aging individuals can become more susceptible and sensitive to side effects such as lightheadedness, confusion, fatigue, constipation, cardiovascular effects, and dry mouth. The central nervous system may be more easily affected in older adults because of changes in the blood-brain barrier and increased side effects of medications. Even if you have taken a medication for years, your body changes as you age and may react differently.

These pages barely scratch the surface of how aging and changes in bodily functions can affect ADME, and you can find many sources that will help you dig deeper into the process. But what is most important is to know that your body changes as you age, and these changes may mean medications should be adjusted or eliminated for safe and effective outcomes.

Thankfully, there are some reliable materials to help providers think carefully about prescribing medications for older adults. Two common guides used by health-care providers are the American Geriatrics Society Beers Criteria [13] and the Screening Tool of Older People's Prescriptions (STOPP).[14] These guides can be used as aids, but providers need to perform a thorough patient evaluation before deciding to start, continue, modify, or stop a medication.

Another noteworthy tool is the STOPPFall (Screening Tool of Older Persons Prescriptions in older adults with high Fall risk). This tool evaluates the likelihood for potential adverse events of a medication, especially if a person is at a high risk of falls.[15]

Potentially Inappropriate Prescribing (PIP)

Potentially inappropriate prescribing (PIP) can cause medications to be prescribed or continued unnecessarily. Increased risk of accidents and emergency visits, adverse drug events, functional decline, and hospitalizations have been related to PIP,[16] which can affect the quality of life and well-being of both patients and their caregivers. Let's look at various scenarios that can be caused or aggravated by PIP.

Medications continued after a health condition has resolved or when a nonpharmacologic approach could have been tried

Individuals may have an episode of depression due to a significant life change, leading a health-care provider to prescribe an antidepressant. A PIP could occur if the antidepressant is never tapered off, if the episode resolves. This type of problematic continuation also occurs when pain and muscle relaxant medications continue to be prescribed even after an injury has healed or physical therapy has resolved an issue. Yet another example, lifestyle changes such as diet and avoiding certain foods that reduce stomach acid could allow for discontinuation of stomach acid products.

Medications or medication combinations continued beyond the time necessary

Multiple blood-thinner (antiplatelet) medications are routinely prescribed after cardiovascular stents are placed due to a blockage to the heart. After six months to a year, only one agent may be necessary, but providers sometimes fail to alter the prescriptions. In another common scenario, proton pump inhibitors initiated for stomach acid and prevention of gastric ulcer during a hospitalization are too often needlessly continued post-hospitalization.

Some medications become unsafe if continued beyond the intended time frame. For example, medications used to increase bone strength, called bisphosphonates, are no longer of benefit after five to ten years of use but instead have an increased risk of causing side effects. Some other medications used for bone density can be used only for a total of two years due to increased risk of side effects. Patients and providers should be aware of these time limits and monitor the length of use.

Medications continued or increased for unlabeled uses or lack of benefit

Gabapentin, a medication used for seizures, is frequently prescribed "off-label" for neuropathic pain. Off-label use means the medication is prescribed for a condition even though there is no FDA approval for its use. However, there may be some case studies or limited scientific evidence-based proof that it works for a particular condition. Gabapentin may be helpful for some patients who use it for neuropathic pain, but it might not be effective for others. Gabapentin is increased to higher doses for treatment benefit but needs to be continually evaluated for effectiveness and appropriateness since it can increase a user's risk of falling.

Over time, your body can build tolerance to some medications, such as benzodiazepines and opioids. When tolerance occurs, healthcare providers may increase doses to achieve the desired benefits. Increasing doses of these medications, which are sometimes inappropriately combined with other meds, can be continued for years in patients even though they may increase falls, dementia, and sedation, especially at higher levels. Patients and providers should be aware that harm can outweigh benefit with some medications.

Medications duplicated with other prescriptions or OTC products

Acetaminophen is a common active ingredient of over-the-counter (OTC) pain, cough and cold, and pain-plus-sleep aids, and it is the same medication as APAP, which is commonly written on prescriptions for a combination of pain or migraine relief. Acetaminophen can cause liver damage if dosed too high. Being aware of all active agents in all medications—prescription or OTC—is important to avoid duplications.

Medications with similar side effects can also cause duplication problems. A medication that is sedating will be additive when combined with another medication that has a sedating side effect, such as an OTC "PM" medication. Taking medications that are sedating can increase the risk of respiratory depression, causing difficulty with breathing and decreased oxygen.

Medications counteracting each other

Some medications have opposite mechanisms of action; that is, they work so differently in the body that the effects of both medications are negated. Donepezil, a medication used for dementia, causes many side effects such as urinary incontinence or overactive bladder, runny nose, and diarrhea (think "wet"). Oxybutynin is used to treat urinary incontinence but can also cause dry eyes, dry nasal passages, and constipation (think "dry"). Oxybutynin may be helpful in taming the inconvenient overactive bladder that donepezil can cause, but it works against the beneficial mechanism of donepezil. Using both negates the benefit of both, especially the treatment of dementia. In addition, many older adults become especially sensitive to oxybutynin, causing them to experience many unwanted side effects.

Medications dosed too aggressively

Poor outcomes may result from overaggressive doses. For example, improper dosages can reduce a patient's blood pressure or blood sugar too much. Or high doses of aspirin may increase the risk of bleeding when a lower dose could be effective and reduce the bleeding risk. High-risk medication treatment for an individual with a limited life expectancy can also be considered overtreatment.

IN REAL LIFE

The story of Mr. Q illustrates the hazards of PIP.

Quetiapine is a medication prescribed for older adults, especially those with dementia, to help with sleep or sleep disturbance. It is an atypical antipsychotic—a newer type of drug used for psychosis—but because it is sedating, it is also used off-label (and potentially inappropriately) to help older adults who have dementia-related moments of disorientation and sleep disturbance.

Mr. Q, who had been diagnosed with Alzheimer's disease, experienced a couple of disoriented nighttime episodes. His wife, who is also his caregiver, mentioned the episodes to Mr. Q's neuropsychologist but assured him her husband was not at all aggressive nor harmful to himself or others and could be redirected without incident. The doctor wrote a prescription for quetiapine for Mr. Q, thinking it would be helpful to reduce these nighttime episodes.

In the meantime, Mr. Q was also experiencing low blood pressure and low blood pressure upon standing, known as orthostatic hypotension. His blood pressure medication had recently been reduced, and he was being monitored to see whether the blood pressure medication could be eliminated. Notably, quetiapine can also cause or add to orthostatic hypotension and can cause heart changes such as arrhythmias. A week after starting quetiapine, Mr. Q was taken to the hospital due to cardiovascular issues.

Mr. Q's hospitalization was most likely precipitated by the quetiapine prescription, which can cause low blood pressure, fainting, and increase falls. It can also cause other cardiovascular side effects, sedation, and dizziness. According to the experts polled for the STOPPFall criteria, 85% to 95% of prescribers would deprescribe the antipsychotic if any of these side effects were present in a patient.[17] Given Mr. Q's condition, quetiapine was most likely inappropriate. Fortunately, he was able to return home after a couple of days.

After Mr. Q returned home, the pharmacist followed up with his doctor to find a safer alternative for the patient.

Other Sources of "Pharm"

Studies show that older adults who take 10 or more medications have worse outcomes on a variety of clinical factors, such as adherence to medications, functional status, cognition, and nutrition.[18] Older adults who took 10 or more meds were more likely to be considered malnourished or at risk of malnourishment due to lower intake of fiber, the B vitamins, and vitamins A, D, E, and K.[19] They were also more likely to have increased intake of fat, sugar, and salt.[20] Some medications reduce appetite, which can become a problem for older adults, even after the individual has taken the medication for a number of years. Some common medications that may cause loss of appetite in older adults and at high doses are fluoxetine and digoxin. Also, many medications can cause stomach upset, constipation, dry mouth, and difficulty swallowing in older adults. It is important to not assume that a loss of appetite is a new symptom of disease or just a sign of getting old when it could very easily be caused by medications. Appetite might improve if the medications are reduced or stopped.

Prolonged overtreatment or overprescribing can also lead to "underprescribing" of needed medications because the patient is already "on so many medications." Instead of considering whether some older medications can be reduced or stopped, a health-care provider may simply choose not to add new medications to the mix, which could deprive an individual of a medication that could be helpful.

Lack of proper medication disposal can also cause problems on the patient's end. The risk of medication mishaps and potential adverse drug reactions rises when people keep old medications. Consider the medications you have around your house. How old are some of them? What is each medication and what is it used for? Do you have old pain relievers or muscle relaxants, leftover antibiotics (I really hope not!), or prescriptions that are a different strength than what you are currently using? Do you still have medications that were stopped because you did not tolerate them well? How about old OTC treatments and herbals? See any potential for confusion here?

Now think about how an older adult who may be confused or forgetful might react to a medicine cabinet like yours—or worse. They may think they need one of the old medications they find in their medicine cabinet, even if their doctors stopped prescribing it years ago. That medication may not be safe or recommended now, or it may interact with other medications the person is currently taking.

Medication Quality and Quality of Life

A study designed to determine the impact of medication quality or appropriateness showed lower medication quality correlates to a lower quality of life.[21] Many patients take inappropriate medications, potentially leading to a poorer quality of life, although the study authors point out that people in the study were rather satisfied with their drug therapy even when it might have been inappropriate or difficult to manage. It's hard to know when you're not living your best life!

Addressing medication appropriateness is important not only for the individual, but also for establishing a health standard. Treatment goals and quality-of-life goals need to be evaluated and monitored when considering medication therapy and quality of treatment. Unfortunately, in many cases, the treatment guidelines, which are relied on heavily for evaluating treatment and the payment system of health-care providers, may not coincide with the quality of prescribing (or deprescribing) medications, especially in older adults.

Medications are certainly wonderful and absolutely have a place in treatment of people of all ages. However, as seen throughout this chapter, medications or combination of medications can sometimes lead to questionable benefits and may even begin to cause harm. Deprescribing or deciding not to prescribe a new medication is a high-quality care option that deserves the same thoughtful attention and documentation that are given to prescribing or continuing medications.

How do patients or caregivers know when it's time to consider deprescribing a medication? Start by empowering yourself through education so you are ready to engage in shared decisions with your prescriber. Then you can begin to renovate your medication list with the tools of deprescribing discussed in Part II.

The ultimate aim of deprescribing is not just to reduce polypharmacy but to improve your health outcomes and quality of life.

Overview of Part I: Overmedicated

- Polypharmacy can be appropriate and beneficial, but it can become an inappropriate and unhelpful overload of medications.
- Medication overload can occur from prescription medications that were never necessary, medications that do not benefit the patient, unnecessary OTC medications, or medications that were once necessary but are no longer needed.
- The more medications a person takes, the higher the risk of an adverse drug event.
- Even "mild" adverse effects, such as dizziness, lightheadedness, nausea, or incontinence, can affect a person's quality of daily living. More severe adverse effects, including delirium, cognitive changes, falls, and bleeding, may lead to life-threatening disabilities and possibly death.
- The culture to prescribe, patient expectations about the benefits of medications, direct-to-consumer advertisements, and marketing to prescribers add to the polypharmacy fire.
- Lifestyle changes may be more beneficial and allow for better quality of life than a full pill box. Multiple medications should not be considered the norm.

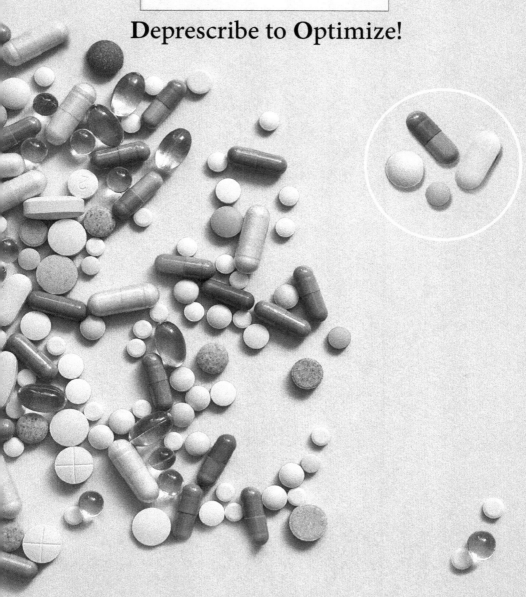

PART II
What Can We DO?
Deprescribe to Optimize!

CHAPTER 4

REMEDY:
REthink the MEDs You take

Introducing the MedStrong
Medication Optimization Plan

DEPRESCRIBING IS A PATH TO OPTIMIZING MEDICATIONS for the individual. It should be a thoughtful process to identify medications that may have more risk than benefit or that may no longer fit the individual's health-care needs or goals. The process of deprescribing is just as valuable to quality health-care practices as is the process of prescribing medications.

When deprescribing, patients or caregivers work with their health-care providers to determine whether a medication may be causing more harm than good and whether that medication can be reduced, changed, or stopped. The patient is monitored and followed after the change, just as when a new medication is started.[22] Deprescribing is a positive, active approach to "patient-centered care" that can help improve health outcomes and reduce adverse drug reactions that could lessen or limit a patient's quality of life.

Deprescribing first appeared in the medical and pharmaceutical literature in 2003.[23] This relatively new idea encompasses stopping medications, reducing medications, or switching to a safer alternative for treatment, and it involves all types of medications. As medications become inappropriate or unnecessary, deprescribing allows them to be withdrawn or changed under the supervision of a health-care provider. Some patients may need to reinstate some medications; however, this has been noted in only a small percentage of cases and does not negate the benefits of deprescribing, which has not been shown to harm the individual.[24]

The concept of deprescribing is taking on new significance as advancements in medical treatments allow people to live longer with multiple medical conditions, which may lead to multiple medications. A component of good prescribing is deprescribing, but our health-care culture is geared more toward starting medications rather than ending them, which can lead to polypharmacy and its associated challenges, which were discussed in previous chapters. Prescribers are inclined to initiate treatment, and patients are often willing to add and continue medications but less supportive of decreasing treatment. Eventually, medication becomes a burden instead of offering beneficial outcomes.[25]

Deprescribing can be a complex and time-consuming process that requires supervised reduction of medications to reduce withdrawal symptoms and improve outcomes that may be associated with polypharmacy. Because deprescribing and prescribing are very similar, they require similar investments of time and energy,[26]and they can provide similar benefits if done well.

Figure 4.1 illustrates the process of prescribing and deprescribing. Do you remember learning to add and subtract using a ruler? If you moved to the right, you were adding and if you moved to the left, you were subtracting. Think of prescribing and deprescribing as learning to add and subtract again. You start at different points on the ruler because each individual is unique. Then you follow a step-by-step approach in either direction, adding or subtracting (prescribing or deprescribing). Of course, you always need to doublecheck your answers (monitor outcomes).

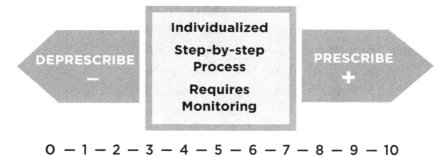

Figure 4.1
Adding and Subtracting Medication

Evidence of the benefits of deprescribing is growing with many medications that could become inappropriate or may be inappropriate from the outset.[27] Deprescribing antihypertensives (blood pressure medication), antipsychotics (for psychosis and agitation in older adults with dementia), and benzodiazepines (for sleep and anxiety) has been reported to reduce patient falls and cardiovascular events and improve cognition and motor function without adverse effects.[28-31]

Deprescribing can also lead to cost containment for individuals, the older adult care community, and the health-care system. Because fewer prescriptions may lead to lower costs and fewer adverse events, falls, and accidents, many individuals and organizations may reap financial benefits of deprescribing practices.

An Eye-Opening Exercise

Part of my advanced pharmacy student rotation at a local hospital calls for pharmacy students to review patient medication lists and find a medication that could be deprescribed. I do not tell the students which patient to choose; it is up to them to review patients on their assigned floor. I have had students tell me they thought I was completely crazy with this assignment: How could they ever pick the correct patient? How dare I not lead them to the patient, at the very least?

However, once they learn about deprescribing, they soon realize most patients on their hospital floor may be taking several medications that may no longer be necessary. Their eyes are opened to a new perspective, and most would agree with one student who said, "I just never really looked at medications this way."

Because I have seen study results about deprescribing and worked with patients whose medications have been decreased by 50%, I am not surprised by what my students find. This reliance on medications may seem alarming to you, but it is a centerpiece of our society's current health-care culture. Consumers are quick to rely on medications, from prescription drugs to over-the-counter (OTC) supplements, and are influenced by the promises from advertisements and the positive reviews from family and friends as to what has worked for them. Providers rely on patient-reported health issues, past experience, and treatment guidelines that lean heavily toward prescribing rather than deprescribing.

Changing the Mind-Set

If you've ever been told, "You will need to take this medicine for the rest of your life," it may seem odd when someone else later tells you, "You no longer need this medication." How would you feel about that kind of change? Elated? Nervous? Uncertain?

Whom would you trust to tell you that a medication you have been taking is no longer necessary? The doctor who prescribed the medication? A specialist? A pharmacist? A nurse, physical therapist, or physician assistant? Would your reaction change depending on which medication is being targeted for discontinuation? Would it matter if it's your medication to treat your blood pressure or your anxiety or your cholesterol levels? How about your medication for seizures if you have not had a seizure in years?

Researchers have found that all these factors matter. Most people are willing to stop medications if their doctor agrees with the move, but their willingness to stop, decrease, or change a drug depends upon the medication. Changes in medications for blood pressure are more acceptable than changes in an antianxiety medication, for example. Though the majority of older people studied thought they were taking a large number of medications, only a small percentage felt they might be taking a medication they no longer needed.[32]

Where to Begin: Medication Optimization Plan

So, now that you know the risks of polypharmacy and the benefits of deprescribing, what should you do next? How do you start the process? And how do you know whether a particular medication should be deprescribed, especially if you do not have a background or expertise in pharmacology or medicine?

Figure 4.2 presents the MedStrong Medication Optimization Plan (MOP) that will help you get started and help you successfully

Figure 4.2

MedStrong Medication Optimization Plan (MOP)
Step-by-Step Deprescribing Guide for the Patient

STEP 1

List all medications.
Fill out the MedStrong Medication List.

STEP 2

Review medication list.
Use the MedStrong Medication List and the MedStrong Question List to formulate questions.

STEP 3

Decide to deprescribe with your provider.
Start the "DO" conversation using the Medstrong Question List.

STEP 4

Make a plan.
Fill out the MedStrong Deprescribing Form.

STEP 5

Monitor, document, follow up.
Use the Medstrong Deprescribing Form and the MedStrong Medication Change Form.

complete the deprescribing process. If you are a caregiver, follow this process to examine the medications of your loved one or patient.

The first step will be discussed in detail in this chapter, where you will also find the MedStrong Medication List. You will find the MedStrong Question List in chapter 5, along with more information about various medications. The MedStrong Deprescribing Form and the MedStrong Medication Change Form are included in chapter 6. All the forms are also included in Appendix A.

STEP 1: List all your medications.
Fill out the MedStrong Medication List.

Write down all the medications you take, whether you take them daily or as needed. Remember the inhalers, eyedrops, nasal sprays, creams, and topicals. Be certain to include prescription and nonprescription medications, over-the-counter (OTC) products, supplements, and herbals—everything counts! Then record the reason you take or use each medication. If you don't know, write that down or put a question mark by the name of the medication. Then look at each medication and the reason you're taking it and ask, "Does this problem still exist? Is the medication I am taking controlling this medical condition?" If you wind up with blank spaces or question marks in your list, those areas should be reviewed first. Here are some helpful hints to rethink the appropriateness of your meds.

- When you are thinking about what nonprescription medicines you have taken, ask yourself these questions: Have I self-treated any ailments with nonprescription medications since my last medical visit? What problems? What did I use?

- Be truthful when making your list! Do you take more or less than what has been prescribed? Then list what you *actually* take, not what your doctor thinks you're taking.

- Write question marks where you are uncertain of the response.

Figure 4.3

MedStrong Medication List

PRESCRIPTION

Name of Prescription Medication and Strength of Dose	How Taken	Reason for Taking	Does the Problem Still Exist?	Is the Medical Condition Controlled?

OVER THE COUNTER

OTC Medication, Supplement, or Herbal and Strength of Dose	How Taken	Reason for Taking	Does the Problem Still Exist?	Is the Medical Condition Controlled?

After recording all your medications and listing why you take each one, check the list to see if you are taking multiple medications for the same reason. If so, it may be appropriate to find out whether all the medications are still needed. Many conditions, such as diabetes, high blood pressure, heart failure, and chronic obstructive pulmonary disease (COPD), typically require multiple medications. However, when treatments change, ask your prescriber if a new medication is being added to the current medications or other medications can be reduced or stopped.

I have seen the effects of miscommunication with health-care providers adding combination inhalers, for example, to a treatment regimen for COPD without the patient clearly understanding that other inhalers need to be stopped. This becomes expensive, and duplicated medications can be harmful, especially with inhalers that contain more than one medication.

When you finish completing your MedStrong Medication List, you will have a comprehensive list of your medications, reasons you are taking each one, and ideas about the effectiveness or potential problems with each of those medicines. With your list in hand, you are ready to begin work on Step 2, reviewing your list and formulating questions about your medications.

CHAPTER 5

Get Your Meds Examined

THROUGHOUT THE YEARS YOU MAY HAVE HEARD, "You need to be your own advocate." Or, from those you care for, "I don't know what I would do without you, I have no idea how to navigate this process." But how do you advocate wisely if you do not have the right tools or resources? How big is your own voice? How can you effectively voice what is important to you?

What do you say when your pharmacist or health-care providers ask, "Do you have any questions?" If you're like most of us, you typically reply, "No."

What is behind that "no"? Many of my patients have told me that "no" really means, "I have no idea what to ask!"

Knowledge is empowering, but knowledge about what questions you can ask to elicit the most helpful information is even more empowering. In this chapter we will explore questions to ask and responses to consider for resistant replies regarding deprescribing. These are not one-time questions; they are the kind of questions that should be asked repeatedly. Our bodies change, our medications most likely change, and our over-the-counter (OTC) products can also change. Keep asking questions to empower yourself, to become a better advocate, and to become a knowledgeable health-care consumer.

Let's get started by reviewing figure 5.1, which is the MedStrong Medication Optimization Plan (MOP) we first encountered in chapter 4. In this chapter, we will tackle Steps 2 and 3.

Figure 5.1

MedStrong Medication Optimization Plan (MOP)
Step-by-Step Deprescribing Guide for the Patient

STEP 1
List all medications.
Fill out the MedStrong Medication List.

STEP 2
Review medication list.
Use the MedStrong Medication List and the
MedStrong Question List to formulate questions.

STEP 3
Decide to deprescribe with your provider.
Start the "DO" conversation using the
Medstrong Question List.

STEP 4
Make a plan.
Fill out the MedStrong Deprescribing Form.

STEP 5
Monitor, document, follow up.
Use the Medstrong Deprescribing Form and the
MedStrong Medication Change Form.

Referring to the comprehensive MedStrong Medication List you completed for Step 1, it is time to consider what questions to ask and how to communicate your concerns to your health-care providers.

STEP 2: Review medication list.
Use MedStrong Medication List and the MedStrong Question List to formulate questions.

After you have completed and reviewed your MedStrong Medication List, the next step is to plan a conversation with your health-care providers to discuss whether you can stop, reduce, or change some of your medications. Consider these questions and concerns that can help open a productive dialogue.[33]

- Is there a good reason why I am taking this medication?
- Is the medication working and providing a needed therapy?
- Is this medication able to provide benefit during my remaining lifespan?

- Is this medication potentially inappropriate now?
- Do I find the dosing and administration of this medication too difficult?
- Would I like to consider stopping this medication? If so, why?
- Could some of the health symptoms I'm experiencing be a side effect of a medication?

As you prepare for your conversation with your doctor or health-care provider, review these questions in the following pages and the rationales for asking them. All of these questions can also be found in the MedStrong Question List (see figure 5.2), which will allow you to highlight the questions you want to be sure to ask in your conversation about optimizing your medications.

Figure 5.2

MedStrong Question List

Check the questions, to ask your health-care providers, that fit your concerns.

Questions to Ask Yourself

☐ Am I having problems paying for all of my prescriptions?

☐ Do I sometimes choose which medicines to take or not take because of affordability issues?

☐ Do I take some or all of my medications differently than how they were prescribed to "stretch them out"? For example, do I take a pill every other day even if it is prescribed to take daily?

Questions to Ask Your Health-Care Provider

☐ Are there any medications that I am currently taking that may no longer be necessary?

☐ Are there any medications that may be dosed too high for my age, health status, kidney function, or with other medications I am taking?

☐ Could one of my health concerns actually be a side effect of a medication?

☐ Are there safer medications I could be taking?

☐ Can any of my medications increase my risk of falls?

☐ Can any combination of these medications increase my risk of falls or increase a risk of bleeding?

Questions to Ask at the Pharmacy

☐ Could I be using an OTC product to treat a side effect of one of my prescription medications?

☐ Is this OTC product okay to take with my current medications and my health conditions?

☐ Are any of my medications potentially being prescribed for a side effect of another prescription (prescribing cascade)?

☐ Could any of my medications increase my risk of falling? If so, which ones?

☐ If I could take fewer medications, which ones should I ask my doctor about possibly stopping?

☐ Am I taking any unnecessary medications?

☐ How long will it take for this medication to start working as it should?

☐ Is this a medication that I need to fill regularly?

☐ When would be the best time of day to take this medication?

☐ Is it possible for you to help me figure out a schedule to take my medications?

Questions to Ask When an Older Adult Is Hospitalized

☐ Could any of my medications—prescription, OTC, herbal, or supplements—have contributed to this condition?

☐ Could my medications have interacted to have caused my hospitalization, such as medications that have additive effects / side effects?

☐ Are there any of my current medications that might be unnecessary or that you think we should discuss with the primary care physician or specialist?

☐ Are there any medications, OTCs, or supplements that may be interacting with blood tests or any other tests or procedures?

Questions to Ask When Being Discharged from the Hospital

☐ Are there changes to my medications or how I should take them?

☐ Are there medications that are similar to medications that I take at home? I do not want to duplicate my medications.

☐ Are there any medications I should no longer take?

☐ How long should I continue taking any new medications? Are some just for a short period of time or just when needed?

My Questions about Specific Concerns or Specific Medications

_____

_____

_____

_____

Questions to Ask Yourself about Your Medications

Before you meet with your health-care providers to discuss your medication concerns, ask yourself some difficult questions. Be truthful with yourself, and then bring the information you learned during your self-examination to your meeting with your doctors. Let your pharmacist, prescribers, and health-care providers know when your medications become too much.

Am I having trouble affording all the medications I take?

Some people do not take medications they need due to affordability issues. Do you choose month to month which medication you pick up at the pharmacy? Are you able to buy nutritious food, or do you have to make a choice between food or medications? Let your doctor know if you are struggling. Many doctors are not aware of how expensive a medication is on your particular insurance plan, and many older adults are embarrassed about their financial standing. Or they may be reluctant to share the costs with the doctor as they think nothing can be done about it.

However, there are several "me too" products that work similarly to address a particular health condition, and insurance plans may vary in how they cover the different products. Be honest about your finances and ask questions about the affordability of various medications—believe me, there are too many insurances for prescribers to be aware of all the nuances and costs. Often prescribers are surprised and have no idea that a medication costs that much for you, so ask if a less expensive medication can do the same thing.

Am I taking any of my medications differently than how they were prescribed?

It can be hard to take every medication as prescribed, especially if regimens are complex or conflict with your schedule, are expensive, or make you feel better if you take it a different way. For example, to better afford a medication, some people will choose to take only half a tablet daily instead of the full tablet that the doctor prescribed. Others may take a medication every other day although it should be taken daily. Some people may take a medication for a chronic condition only when they are having symptoms, although the medication should be taken every day to keep the condition under control.

Again, be truthful with your prescribers. Let them know if you are not taking the medication as intended. Otherwise, a provider may think a medication is not working well when the problem could be that you are not taking the full dose of the prescription. That could lead to a higher dosage or to new medications.

If you explain your problem to your prescriber, you might be surprised at the different arrangements that can be made. Maybe you don't need to take the pill, or it could be switched to something else, or perhaps the dose may need to be changed. Understanding the situation allows the provider to make informed decisions.

In addition to considering which questions to ask, you should also consider which questions to ask in a particular situation. The process may look slightly different depending on the health-care setting, so let's examine a few common scenarios.

Questions to Ask a Health-Care Provider

It can be intimidating to start a conversation with your doctor or other health-care provider, especially if you want to ask them about deprescribing. You can open the conversation by telling your provider that you want to look at your medications because you want to take a proactive approach to reduce your risk of poor outcomes as you age. Mention preventing falls and cognition deficits or any other concern you may have and then ask the questions you have prepared. Let's look at some questions you could use to start that discussion and consider what responses you might get.

Are there any medications I am currently taking that may no longer be necessary?

This question takes a pretty direct approach, and it may make your doctor a little defensive. So, don't be too surprised if you receive a quick response along the lines of, "No, everything is fine that you are taking."

Deprescribing is a thoughtful process, and you really deserve a more thoughtful answer than "No, you are all set." It's going to be a much better conversation if you hear, "You really do need all of these medications for your current conditions, do you have a concern about something?" Big difference in these responses.

Don't give up if you do get a too-quick, too-dismissive response initially. Consider following up with one of the next questions.

Is this [specific medication] still necessary?

Do you really need the antacid / acid suppressant, pain reliever, or bone density product you have been taking for five years now? Instead of asking your doctor to review your entire medication list and consider what could be stopped, ask about a particular medication.

Read chapter 7 and consider if you are taking any of the medications listed there and whether they might be causing any problems. Be specific about your questions and why you think it might be time to discontinue, reduce, or substitute that medication.

Are there safer medications I could be taking?

Safety is so important with medications. Let your doctor know if you are experiencing health issues that could be caused by your medications. You may take many diabetes medications but have recently been experiencing more low blood sugar episodes, known as hypoglycemia. Ask your doctor if reducing your diabetes medications could help reduce your hypoglycemic episodes.

Or you can ask if you could switch to a product that still treats a condition but has fewer potential side effects. Many medication families have similar types of medications that vary in side effects. Finding the right medication for you can be beneficial.

Could it be a side effect?

Review your MedStrong Medication List to consider whether you are experiencing new or intensified side effects of your medications, and then relay your concerns to your doctor. How can you tell if you are experiencing any side effects? You may just think you're not feeling well instead of realizing that some of your problems could be caused by your medications. Think long and hard about how often you experience headaches, or feel tired or achy, or fall. Are your eyes dry? Are you always thirsty? Do you feel confused, have "brain fog" or "senior moments"? These symptoms may be due not to "just age," but to medication working differently than it did years ago.

Do you sometimes get dizzy or lightheaded when you stand up from your chair? Maybe you're experiencing a medication side effect. Some blood pressure medications may cause lightheadedness and/or dizziness when you change positions, such as moving from sitting to standing. This can be due to a drop in blood pressure, also known as orthostatic hypotension. Some people may be experiencing the drop in blood pressure without feeling it, but they may still be at an increased risk of falling or fainting. Antidepressants, pain medications, or medications for benign prostatic hyperplasia (BPH) also cause this lowering of blood pressure; taking more than one of these kinds of medicines might cause the side effects to be stronger.

Are any of your symptoms listed as side effects for any of your medications? Talk to your doctor about your concerns. Most of us expect that a new symptom needs to be treated, but few of us consider that *stopping* a medication might alleviate an issue, especially if we have been taking a medication with no apparent problems for a long time.

I have been relying on over-the-counter products to (explain the reason). Could I be treating a side effect of one of my prescriptions?

Let your doctor know if you have needed to self-medicate with OTC products; for example, you have been using natural tears, or medicine for constipation, or headache pain relief. Perhaps you are actually treating the side effects of one of your prescription drugs. Remember, even if you have been taking a medication for years, you may develop new side effects because your body is changing.

Can any of my medications increase my risk of falls?

Falls can be caused or compounded by medications, particularly those that may change heart rhythm or heart rate, cause dizziness, unsteadiness, confusion, or drowsiness. Older adults are frequently taking more than one medication that could increase the risk of falls, which could lead to an additive effect. Be certain your medications are correctly dosed and ask your provider to switch or reduce your fall-risk medications before you take a tumble.

Can any combination of these medications increase my risk of bleeding? Would that be a concern if I fell?

Many medications, especially those that work to prevent blood clots, can increase your risk of bleeding. Aspirin and OTC NSAIDs, such as ibuprofen and naproxen, can also increase the risk of bleeding. If you have been taking any medications that can increase your risk of bleeding, a fall might cause internal bleeding, which would be as concerning as a wound that does not stop bleeding. You might be surprised at some of the medications and supplements that can increase bleeding, such as garlic, omega-3, and some medications used for depression and anxiety.

Is it possible that I could feel better if I stopped a medication?

Your doctors may not spend a lot of time thinking about how

your medications make you feel. Instead, they are evaluating as to whether the medication seems to be keeping your disease or illness under control. So, it's up to you let your health-care providers know when you're not feeling as good as you would like. Deprescribing a medication may make you feel better than you would if you added something new. Health-care providers not only need to ensure they are treating conditions or ailments but also to have patients feel the best they possibly can. Your calm questions can help the provider focus more on your feelings and success stories.

Could a medication I am taking make me feel [this way]?

Review chapter 7 and note how many medications can cause unwanted side effects, and how drug-disease interactions can cause a medication to worsen another condition. As with the previous question, this one can help you focus your doctor's attention on how you feel. It can also let the provider know that you are willing to give up a medicine if it will make you feel better.

Questions to Ask at the Pharmacy

Pharmacists are available to counsel on prescription medications and non-prescription selections, potential drug interactions or duplications, and best timing to take your medications. Pharmacists review medications that are ordered, provide instructions for use, provide insurance information for coverage, and counsel patients on their medication and vaccinations. Pharmacists are your first and last line of defense and are readily accessible to provide health-care information. You can ask your pharmacist questions similar to those you ask your other providers.

Questions to Ask When an Older Adult Is Hospitalized

An illness or accident that results in hospitalization can be a frightening and confusing time for anyone. But it can be an ideal time to ask health-care providers some questions about medications.

You may need to ask questions about your own meds, or you may be gathering information about a family member or someone that you are caring for. Whatever the situation, use these questions—adapted to your situation—to start a productive discussion.

Could any of my medications—prescription, OTC, herbal, or supplements—have contributed to my condition?

Discuss with your doctors whether your kidney function has changed, even temporarily, due to an acute change in your health. Reduced kidney function changes can cause medication to not be eliminated from your system efficiently, potentially causing drastic health problems that can lead to a hospitalization

Has there been a change in my electrolytes due to a medication or dehydration? Could a medication be too potent for me at my age? Could changes in my body and my medication make me feel more lethargic, weak, and confused? While you are discussing these questions with your health-care providers, also think about what you've been taking that your doctors might not know about. Did you recently pick up or order a new OTC or herbal product? Or did you recently start or stop a medication? If so, mention it to your providers when you have this discussion.

In the hospital, you may have the chance to ask these questions to multiple health-care providers, including specialists, pharmacists, and physical therapists. Collect information and opinions from as many people as you can. And don't stop when you're released; ask again when you receive follow-up care or when you pick up your new prescriptions.

Are any of my medications unnecessary? Are there any medications I should bring to the attention of my primary care physician or specialist?

Many medications are prescribed for chronic conditions that may not be related to your hospital stay, and hospitalists will rarely change medications prescribed by other doctors, especially if they do not pertain to the exact reason you are in the hospital. But you should take advantage of having several health-care providers in a hospital setting who can give you their opinions about your health and medications. Ask, in their opinion, if all of your medications are still necessary, appropriate, and safe.

Also be sure to ask questions about any new medications that are prescribed while you are in the hospital. Should they be continued indefinitely? Will your general practitioner be informed about the new medications and about any time or dosage limits?

More Conversation Starters

You've seen several ideas in the past few pages about how to start deprescribing conversations in certain settings. Here are a few more ideas, which have been adapted from an article in the *American Family Physician* [34] These guidelines were originally written to help health-care providers open conversations about deprescribing. But they have been adapted here to help show patients how to open conversations with their physicians.

Exploring options

- How important is it that I take [name your medication]?
- It is important to me that I continue to take medications I need, but I would be willing to stop some medications if I could.
- Can we decide if I really need to take all these medications?
- I would like to try a trial of stopping or reducing [name your medication] to see how it goes.
- If the medication(s) could be causing side effects, could we try to stop or reduce it/them to see if it helps?

Benefit versus risk

- If we decide to reduce or stop [name your medication], how might I feel? How will I know whether I am benefitting from the change or if I need to restart the medicine?

- I am taking several medications now. I would like to review these regularly to be sure that each one is still a benefit and to check for side effects.

_____

_____

- I understand that medication side effects can add up. Do my medications have some similar side effects that could be making me tired, constipated, forgetful, fall? [Fill in your specific condition here.]

_____

_____

- I read that as we age medications we have taken successfully for years may become more of a harm than a benefit and no longer needed. Are some medications I take a concern? I'm wondering about [mention any meds you have taken for a long period of time].

_____

_____

_____

- I heard some medications are needed only for a short period of time, but it seems like I have been taking [name your medication] for quite some time.

_____

_____

_____

Talking Deprescribing with Your Loved Ones

Caregivers can sometimes talk directly to health-care providers about deprescribing, but they usually have to first broach the topic directly with their loved one. How do family members or caregivers bring up deprescribing when they fear their loved one will be resistant to the idea?

- Explain that deprescribing should be a thoughtful process and a way to optimize their medications.
- Explain that the change does not have to be set in stone. The patient will be monitored to see how they feel when medications are reduced, switched, or stopped.
- Celebrate them for being proactive in their health.

Jane Brody, a personal health columnist for the *New York Times*, recently wrote about a pharmacist's 87-year-old mother, who suffered through a series of emergency department visits and hospitalizations, all of which were likely linked to inappropriate prescriptions, according to her daughter.[35] Brody included in her article a list of questions that should be asked before accepting and starting a new prescription. Getting answers to these questions is especially important for older adults.

- Am I experiencing a symptom that could be a side effect of one of my medications?
- Is this new med being used to treat a side effect?
- Is there a safer med available than the one I am taking?
- Could I take a lower dose of this medicine?
- Do I need to take this med at all?

Unfortunately, I know many people have suffered through experiences like the one Brody described, and as seen in her article, this can even happen to family members of those in health care. I have heard physicians tell similar stories about overmedicated relatives.

As I said at the beginning of this chapter, "You need to be your own advocate." Use the information you've found in this chapter to empower yourself and ask the questions that will help you optimize your medications.

But don't expect that one conversation or one medication change will be sufficient. Follow-up is needed any time medications are adjusted. You can't make changes blindly, because not all changes are good changes and not all changes last forever. That's what will be examined in the next chapter.

STEP 3. Decide to deprescribe with your provider.
Start the "DO" conversation using the MedStrong Question List.

Now that you have your questions and have begun the "DO" (Deprescribe to Optimize) conversation with your health-care providers, you are ready for the next step: deciding with your providers to deprescribe if necessary. This part of the process is similar to Step 2, as it involves more conversation with your doctor. But it's different because it focuses on specific targeted medications to consider in your particular case. Shared decision-making is the crucial factor in this step.

As in Step 2, the DO process may look slightly different depending on the health-care setting.

Deprescribing in the Primary-Care Setting

Although deprescribing is most often undertaken today in end-of-life, long-term-care settings, many people could benefit from the DO process if it were undertaken much earlier. And it is usually most successful when undertaken with the advice of a primary care provider or general practitioner[36] and the expertise of a pharmacist. Your primary care provider should be able to easily access your full medical profile, disease diagnoses, notes from specialists, and prescription records. Ideally, all practitioners—including specialists and hospitalists—should be involved in deprescribing, but your primary care setting is a good place to start.

Your provider should know about all your prescription medication, but it is also important to be honest about all the OTC medicines, supplements, or herbal products that you take, as all of these products can affect the performance of your prescription medications. Make an appointment with your provider and let them know you want to discuss your medications and whether all continue to be necessary and appropriate. Be prepared to show your provider your MedStrong Medication List and to raise the questions or concerns from your MedStrong Question List.

Also be prepared to follow any plan your provider recommends and to schedule follow-up visits to provide feedback on any positive or negative consequences.

The Royal Pharmaceutical Society outlines four principles for providers to optimize medications within a patient-centered approach to improve outcomes and align measurement and monitoring parameters[37]

Principle 1. Understand the patient's perspective, views, and preferences.

Principle 2. Assess the evidence base and cost effectiveness of treatments.

Principle 3. Ensure medicine safety.

Principle 4. Optimize medications as part of routine practice. Even though this list is written primarily for the provider, it's easy to consider the same principles from a patient point of view.

Principle 1. What are your views regarding your medications and preferences?

Principle 2. Are you able to afford your medications as prescribed and are they effective?

Principle 3. Do you feel well and strong? Have you fallen recently? Do you sometimes feel dizzy or unsteady?

Principle 4. Ask about your medications regularly; don't wait for a fall, a hospitalization, or accident to ask about making a change.

Asking about your medications regularly with your primary care provider can cultivate a better relationship with the provider and make you more confident about the medications you are taking. Take this approach with all of your caregivers, including physicians, nurses, physician assistants, pharmacists, and all other health-care providers you see.

Unless you introduce the idea of deprescribing, physicians or other prescribers may be reluctant to bring it up until you or someone you care for is facing limited life expectancy, cognitive impairment, or pill burden. I say, why wait for all that? Why not eliminate medications that can potentially affect cognition before they actually do significant damage? Why keep thinking it's "normal" to add more medications to your already long list of medications without reviewing to see if you can discontinue some? Ask your provider to take the time to consider these issues with you.

Deprescribing in the Hospital Setting

A hospitalization—especially as the result of a fall or other accident—may offer an ideal opportunity to discuss the DO process for you or someone you are caring for. Many patients who are admitted to the hospital for a fall take medications that can increase the risk of a fall.[38]

Hospital care providers, including pharmacists, may consider deprescribing to reduce risk of future falls—especially if the patient or patient's caregiver introduces the topic.

A hospital stay should always indicate that medication reviews are warranted, and action to deprescribe should be welcomed to reduce further risk. Patients should not necessarily be sent home on more medications than they were taking unless a thorough review of current medications is performed. So be ready to speak up for yourself or the person you care for. Ask whether any of your current medications could have contributed to the accident or illness that made your hospital stay necessary. Ask whether your hospital care team is recommending new medications. If so, are the new medicines likely to interact negatively with any of your current prescriptions? Does your hospital team think you could discontinue any of your current medications?

Deprescribing in Long-Term Care

People in long-term care tend to have multiple conditions that make them unable to care for themselves, so they must rely on loved ones and caregivers to advocate for them. Caregivers should meet regularly with health-care providers to review medications and determine if deprescribing is possible.

Family members or other patient advocates may not realize that there are guidelines for many medications and that pharmacists are contracted to review patient charts monthly on behalf of insurance providers. If you are serving as a caregiver for someone in long-term care, ask to discuss these guidelines with that person's care team.

Don't be surprised if the care team suggests deprescribing dementia medications or other drugs, as they may now pose more risks than benefits. Some family members worry that discontinuing dementia medications could further worsen a loved one's condition or lead to behavioral or mood changes, but there is no conclusive evidence to confirm these fears. However, there is good evidence to show that discontinuing such medications can reduce side effects such as fainting, hip fracture, arrhythmia, urinary incontinence, and diarrhea.[39]

As a caregiver, you may also be called on to make difficult decisions to deprescribe or stop medications that treat chronic conditions when it is time for your loved one to transition to hospice or comfort care. I remember reviewing medications for my father as his dementia worsened and a new diagnosis of cancer prevailed. I distinctly remember thinking, "This is what we teach and know, in pharmacy and in health care, that certain medications are stopped at this time." Even so, I had to take a deep breath before agreeing with the prescriber as to the plan of action. Although it was a hard decision to make, I knew it was best to keep my father comfortable but not treat his chronic health conditions any longer.

The Goal of Shared Decision-Making

Deprescribing should be a process that is shared between patients, caregivers, and a team of health-care providers. There are many factors to explore when embarking on deprescribing options, including awareness, psychology, communication, and decision-making. Recognizing the factors that can hinder or promote the process can give you a head start on the DO road. Each factor brings its challenges, whether you are the patient, caregiver, or health-care provider.

Learning that options to your extensive medication list exist can be eye-opening—both for you and your health-care providers.[40] Prime opportunities to review your deprescribing options arise during times of transition from one health-care setting or provider to another, when new symptoms appear, or when high-risk medications are identified. Ideally, though, medications should be reviewed regularly. Don't wait for a fall, accident, side effect, or hospitalization to initiate a discussion about your medication with your health-care provider.

Emotional and mental biases can make it more difficult for either patient or provider to initiate a deprescribing process. The cognitive bias that favors "status quo" may make you reluctant to ask for a medication review, especially if you have been taking a particular medication for years. That same bias may make a prescriber reluctant to review medications that seem to be working, because they don't want to "fix something that is not broken." Clinical inertia occurs when patients and/or providers know about the potential advantages of deprescribing but do not act on that knowledge.[41] This in turn leads to omission bias as a tendency to not take action leading to inaction and unwillingness to change in future situations.[42] Sometimes multiple attempts to initiate a deprescribing process must be made by either patient or provider to overcome these biases.

A basic level of health literacy is needed when you are discussing medication issues with your health-care provider. You do not need to have a doctor's level of understanding of pharmaceuticals, but you will reap many benefits from learning basic information about your health and treatment options. A knowledge of numeracy also is needed in these conversations. Brush up on the concepts of quantity, days' supply, number of times per day a medication is prescribed, and insurance costs.

Most important of all is the willingness to ask questions and to admit any confusion. Patients should always be willing to say, "I'm not sure I understand. Can you explain in a different way?" Never hesitate to ask a prescriber to repeat information or to write down instructions so you can review later. You can always ask if you can repeat something back to make certain you are clear on the information you are receiving. Providers should check for understanding by asking a patient to repeat back information or instructions or to explain understanding of a concept.

If you are a patient or caregiver, know what you want and be ready to speak up for yourself! Your strong preference may be for your doctor to make the final decision—if that's true, then be sure to say so. Ask questions if you're not sure. You might ask your doctor, "If you were me, what would you do?" Once your health-care providers know what you prefer, a shared decision can be made. Of course, decisions should not be set in stone; they should be reviewed, monitored, and revisited throughout the health-care process.

Your goals as a patient or caregiver may be very different from the goals of a prescriber who is relying on medication protocols for a patient or a specific disease state. A patient with multiple health issues who is diagnosed with cancer may have different treatment goals than an otherwise healthy patient who is diagnosed with the same cancer. A patient's goals may also change and evolve slowly over time, especially as they age.

Get input from your whole team of care providers and be ready to defend your preferences and to demand that your doctor hear you out. One older woman spoke with me regarding her husband's medications and then tried to bring up her—and my—concerns at his next medical appointment. The doctor brushed off the concerns, stating, "Pharmacists only care about side effects." If you find yourself in such a scenario, be prepared to push back. You could reply, "I have a lot of respect for this professional. I think they are trying to look out for me and my continued well-being. Could we explore options?"

Fortunately, not all doctors respond in such cavalier ways to patients' medication concerns. I have seen nurse practitioners, geriatricians, social workers, and pharmacists working together to optimize a patient's medications by listening to each other and discussing options. I say, "Bravo!" to this process.

CHAPTER 6

Flip the Scrip

YOU HAVE USED YOUR MEDSTRONG MEDICATION LIST to record all your medications and your MedStrong Question List to note your questions or concerns. (Find the MedStrong Medication List in chapter 4 and the MedStrong Question List in chapter 5.) You reviewed and formulated questions for your doctors and pharmacists and engaged with them in (hopefully) productive conversations. You have thought about what over-the-counter (OTC), herbal, and supplement products you take and have pondered whether a problem you are trying to treat could be a side effect of a medication you have been taking. You have considered why you started taking each of your medications and made sure you have solid reasons to continue them, and you have carefully thought about how aging can change your body and the way you react to your medications. You've asked yourself whether you're feeling weak, tired, or dizzy just because you're getting older or if those problems could be related to a lifestyle choice or medication you are taking.

You have learned how to start—and continue—a conversation with your doctor and pharmacist and other health-care providers about your medications. You learned how to share your goals for your life as a way to introduce the deprescribe to optimize (DO) process. You talked with your health-care providers about whether any of your medications may be unnecessary, inappropriate, or excessive.

In other words, you've done lots of work so far. Don't stop! Now is the time to "flip the scrip" and act on those discussions. You should now be ready for Step 4 of the MedStrong Medication Optimization Plan (MOP). (See figure 6.1.)

Figure 6.1

MedStrong Medication Optimization Plan (MOP)
Step-by-Step Deprescribing Guide for the Patient

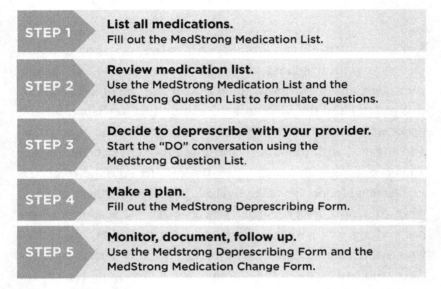

STEP 1
List all medications.
Fill out the MedStrong Medication List.

STEP 2
Review medication list.
Use the MedStrong Medication List and the MedStrong Question List to formulate questions.

STEP 3
Decide to deprescribe with your provider.
Start the "DO" conversation using the Medstrong Question List.

STEP 4
Make a plan.
Fill out the MedStrong Deprescribing Form.

STEP 5
Monitor, document, follow up.
Use the Medstrong Deprescribing Form and the MedStrong Medication Change Form.

Use the MedStrong Deprescribing Form (see figure 6.2) to help keep your plans straight and to help you evaluate your results. You can use this process for yourself or for a family member or client if you are a caregiver.

STEP 4. Make a plan.
Fill out the MedStrong Deprescribing Form.

Your health-care provider should document medications that have been deprescribed, but it's also a good idea for you to keep your own written records to help you remember details about the decisions you made. Jot down notes about why a medication was reduced, changed, or stopped and describe how the change will occur. You also want to record how you feel during the process. The MedStrong Deprescribing Form provided in this chapter will help you document the decisions and the monitoring process.

You may also want to keep a journal or calendar to document the changes and the dates of the changes. Some hospitals and doctor offices may provide a list of medications to continue, medications that have changed, and medications to stop when changes are made to your prescriptions. Be certain you review these printouts and medication lists carefully.

Use a MedStrong Deprescribing Form for each medication change and be certain you are recording the correct medication. I know this sounds crazy, but there are so many similar sounding medications that you want to be certain you and your doctor or pharmacist are talking about the same medication. Don't abbreviate the name of the medicine or product or use shorthand or nicknames on your form—be very specific.

Use the form to record the decision to stop, change, or reduce the medication. Be certain you are clear on this step. Are you able to stop taking the med immediately or does the medication need to be tapered? Record the date you were given these instructions and the date you began the change.

This is also a good time to ask whether you are taking any medications as part of a "prescribing cascade." Were any of your medications prescribed to treat the side effects of a medication that is being deprescribed? Ask your health-care provider whether other medications may no longer be needed if you stop a particular prescription.

STEP 5. Monitor, document, follow up.
Use the MedStrong Deprescribing Form and MedStrong Medication Change Form.

Next, start monitoring the changes in your health and body and record the relevant information on the MedStrong Deprescribing Form. Monitoring and follow-up help close the loop on the deprescribing process to ensure that the changes are helpful and not harmful. Will you need to check lab results in order to monitor your health conditions after you stop or change a particular medication? Record that here. Do you need to keep an eye on a vital sign and log the results for your follow-up appointment? Record that here.

Also, it is important to record how you feel, so be certain to keep a daily log to monitor any changes. If you are not doing well or have some problems with the change, record how you feel and review with your physician. If you feel better, record that too. And be sure to record if you don't feel any different, which could be considered a successful outcome for this deprescribing process.

After deprescribing has occurred, be certain to update your medication list! You can use the Medstrong Medication Change Form shown in figure 6.3 to update your list. See figure 6.4 for an example.

As you have learned in this chapter and throughout this book, having a clear plan and realistic expectations will help you address any fear or reservations you may have about stopping or changing a medication. Use the MedStrong MOP and its relevant forms to help navigate this process.

The next chapter, "What's in Your Pill Box?" explores various medications and scenarios that patients have experienced; highlighting how any medication that can be beneficial to one person can impose risk or harm on another. Let's continue the journey to optimize medications for the best outcomes.

Figure 6.2

MedStrong Deprescribing Form

Medication: _____ Date: _____

Why is this medication being deprescribed? _____

Deprescribe Instructions: _____

☐ Changed to: _____

☐ Reduced to: _____

☐ Stopped: Date: _____

Taper: Yes ☐ No ☐

If yes, taper instructions: _____

_____

Monitor: _____

☐ Labs: _____ Date: _____

☐ Check: _____ and keep a log.

(Examples: blood pressure, heart rate, blood glucose, weight)

Date: _____ Time: _____ Results: _____

How do I feel?:

☐ No different: _____

☐ Not so good because: _____

☐ Better, I notice that: _____

Follow-up with:

Name of health care provider: _____

Phone number: _____

Date of next appointment: _____

Figure 6.3 **MedStrong Medication Change Form**

Medication and Strength	How Many, How Often	Prescribed by	Date/Year Started	Still Taking?	Date Med Stopped or Changed	Medication Restarted or Changed, Why?

Figure 6.4 **Sample of MedStrong Medication Change Form**

Medication and Strength	How Many, How Often	Prescribed by	Date/Year Started	Still Taking?	Date Med Stopped or Changed	Medication Restarted or Changed, Why?
Amlodipine 10 mg	1 daily	Dr. H	Jan 2020	N	Feb 2022	Decreased (ankle edema)
Amlodipine 5 mg	1 daily	Dr. H	Feb 2022	Y		

CHAPTER 7

What's in Your Pill Box?

T HE FIRST STEP in the MedStrong Medication Optimization Plan (MOP) is to list all your medications. As you continue through the process of formulating questions, discussing your medications with your providers, and eventually working through the deprescribe to optimize (DO) steps, certain types of medications should get priority attention, especially if they are being taken by an older adult. These types of medications include antipsychotics, statins, antihypertensives, benzodiazepines, proton pump inhibitors (PPIs), anticholinergics, sedatives, opioids, and nonsteroidal anti-inflammatory drugs (NSAIDs), including aspirin and COX-2 inhibitors, such as celecoxib.

Whether you are a provider who prescribes these medications on a daily basis or a patient who can barely pronounce some of these terms, recognize that all medications have their limitations and that some can become especially problematic for older adults. This chapter examines some common medications and describes some not-so-uncommon patient scenarios to help health-care providers, patients, and caregivers understand how a once-beneficial medication can become unnecessary, inappropriate, or excessive.

The medications or family groups of medication are presented in alphabetical order, and all drugs are listed by their generic drug names. Many of the scenarios described in this chapter may remind you of your own medication stories or may offer unexpected insight into how a medication may be affecting you or someone you know.

Although many common medications and scenarios are mentioned, this chapter does not provide an exhaustive list of medications or reasons for concern. Any medication, prescription or nonprescription, can become potentially unnecessary or harmful depending upon your health status, chronic health conditions, pharmacodynamics (what the drug does to the body), and pharmacokinetics (what the body does to the drug). See appendix A for the full chart of medication families and similar products, provided throughout this chapter. Comparing names of similar medications may help you navigate your own scenarios.

Anticholinergics ("anti-coal-in-er-jix")

Anticholinergic medications are used for Parkinson's, urinary incontinence, overactive bladder, stomach spasms, nausea, vomiting, and chronic obstructive pulmonary disease (COPD). Many additional medications, including muscle relaxants, older first-generation antihistamines (used for allergies and sleep), medications used for depression and anxiety, and antipsychotics also have anticholinergic properties or side effects.

The following is just a small list of commonly used medications that fall into the category of anticholinergics. An anticholinergic burden calculator is also provided under Resources at the end of the book. Note, there are several anticholinergic burden calculators, indicating this is an important issue. It is. Especially as we age.

Anticholinergics used for	
urinary incontinence	oxybutynin, solifenacin, tolterodine
COPD	aclidinium, ipratropium, tiotropium, umeclidinium
parkinsonism	benztropine
stomach spasm	dicyclomine, hyoscyamine
motion sickness, nausea, vomiting	scopolamine

Anticholinergics should be prime suspects in a search for potentially inappropriate medications. They can be very drying, causing dry eyes, dry nasal passages, dry mouth, difficulty swallowing, and urinary retention—that's why they are frequently used as incontinence medications. Other side effects include fast heart rate, confusion, and balance issues that can increase the risk of falls.

These effects are so concerning that anticholinergic burden calculators have been developed to calculate a total burden score. The number of medications reported as having these potential effects and the level of potential danger can vary from one calculator to the next; however, all serve as helpful means of quantifying a potential risk. It is best to choose safer medications that have no to low anticholinergic activity or to deprescribe medications that may no longer be necessary.

In the study "Assessing Risks of Polypharmacy Involving Medications with Anticholinergic Properties,"[43] anticholinergic calculators were found to vary in their details, but all proved to be beneficial in calculating risk for poor outcomes, including cognition, dementia, delirium, mortality, cardiovascular events, and admissions for falls and fractures. Regardless of which calculator you use, the goal is to reduce and limit the anticholinergic score to help reduce poor outcomes. The anticholinergic burden can affect younger adults too; this is not just for the oldest old and frailest old, though they are very much impacted.

In fact, concerns are growing over using anticholinergic agents to treat older adults, as they have been shown to increase risk of falls and hospitalizations, reduce function, and cause changes in mental status.[44] Though these dangers are recognized as potentially inappropriate, little change has been made in prescribing anticholinergic agents to older adults, especially in acute-care settings. A study reviewed the anticholinergic burden for patients over 65 years old who were admitted to a hospital for falls, fracture, or altered mental status. These patients were evaluated and followed for anticholinergic burden score from admission to discharge. Patients whose anticholinergic burden increased or stayed the same were more likely to be readmitted to the hospital within 30 days. The oldest group of patients, those 85 years and older, were also more likely to have an increased anticholinergic burden during their hospital stay than the other patients. Lack of deprescribing and additional prescribing are both areas of concern, especially when anticholinergic burden scores remain the same or even increase, as this causes increased risk of side effects for the patient.

Health-care providers, patients, and caregivers should review new medications—especially any prescriptions begun during a hospital stay—and ask whether these can contribute to the anticholinergic burden. It's also a good idea to look at medications you already take to calculate the risk of anticholinergic burden. You can use the anticholinergic calculator referenced under Resources at the end of the book. Use the template provided in figure 7.1 to discuss anticholinergic concerns with your prescriber. A score greater than three should be reviewed for potential deprescribing.

Figure 7.1

MedStrong Anticholinergic Burden Scoring Sheet

Date: _____ Scale Used: _____

Medication	Listed on anticholinergic scale? Y/N	Score
	Number of medications Y =	Total:

Antidepressants

Antidepressants are used for many types of depression. These medications can also overlap and be used for other mental health issues including anxiety, obsessive-compulsive disorder, and posttraumatic stress disorder. Below is a list of some common antidepressants.

Antidepressants	
SSRIs	fluoxetine, paroxetine, sertraline, citalopram, escitalopram
SNRIs	duloxetine, venlafaxine
TCAs	amitriptyline, nortriptyline
Others	bupropion, mirtazapine, trazodone

Antidepressants and other medications used primarily for mental health treatment are a particular source of uncertainty for deprescribing. It can be difficult to know whether a person's depression has improved because of the medication or their depression has improved because of other factors. Prescribers and patients also may be concerned with potential withdrawal symptoms and leery of recurrence or relapse.

However, a patient who continues to take antidepressants needlessly can increase the risk of side effects, such as sedation, sleep disturbance, confusion, drop in blood pressure upon standing (orthostatic hypotension), blurred vision, dementia, tremors or other movement disorders, low sodium levels, fractures, drug-drug interactions, and cardiovascular changes, including arrhythmias. Many of these side effects can increase the risk of falls,[45] but depression can also increase the risk of falls. Talk about a "Catch-22"—both depression and antidepressants can increase the risk of falls!

There are many types of antidepressants, and some may be more likely to cause certain side effects than others. Therefore, even if you and your doctor decide treatment is necessary, discuss if it might be possible to switch to a more appropriate medication that would have fewer side effects and more benefits for you. Various families of antidepressants, especially tricyclic antidepressants (TCAs) such as amitriptyline, have a very high side-effect profile for orthostatic hypotension, cardiovascular side effects, daytime drowsiness, confusion, movement disorders, and sedation.

Selective serotonin reuptake inhibitors (SSRIs) tend to cause more stomach upset, hyponatremia (low sodium), and cardiovascular effects than other antidepressants. Other antidepressants also have their risks. Bupropion is known for increasing seizure risk, mirtazapine for sedation and orthostatic hypotension effects, and trazodone for imbalance and sedation problems.

Too often, when patients are taking antidepressants, multiple antidepressants may be added while none are deprescribed. The side effects become additive and can cause geriatric syndromes such as cognitive impairment, falls, and fatigue, to name only a few potential problems. If you and your provider decide you should keep taking an antidepressant, it is important to reevaluate whether you need more than one type. It's also important to regularly assess your continued need and to pay attention to whether you are suffering from side effects, especially as your body changes over time.

Antipsychotics

Antipsychotics are medications used to treat delirium, disorientation, paranoia, schizophrenia, and bipolar disorders. These medications can be used short-term (episodically) or long-term.

Antipsychotics	
Second Generation	aripiprazole, clozapine, iloperidone, lurasidone, olanzapine, paliperidone, pimavanserin, quetiapine, risperidone, ziprasidone
First Generation	haloperidol

Quetiapine and aripiprazole are FDA-approved for bipolar disorder and schizophrenia, but they are also commonly used as an off-label therapy in older adults for agitation associated with dementia. Quetiapine is also frequently seen on medication lists to be taken in the evening to improve sleep. Many products are used in this type of off-label fashion, but these medications, due to their potential side effects, should be reserved as alternative therapy. After a patient—especially an older adult—uses one of these medications for a few months, the patient or caregiver should review the medication with the provider to determine if it can be reduced or deprescribed, particularly if the acute episode that was the catalyst for the prescription has resolved.

Antipsychotics can lead to falls in the middle of the night due to the potential for orthostatic hypotension, a drop in blood pressure that occurs when a person changes from a lying or sitting position to a standing position. These same medications can cause cardiovascular changes, resulting in potential arrhythmias, and can reduce cognitive function. Furthermore, if the medication is not alleviating the agitation or is causing worsening of symptoms, increasing the dose is a questionable strategy. I have unfortunately seen this occur, especially with patients who have Alzheimer's because it is difficult to treat their agitation and there are limited options available to do so.

Sometimes medications need to be used or continued even when there are concerns about personal safety—especially in situations when safety of others may be threatened. This is part of the risk-versus-benefit analysis that needs to be weighed in those with mental health conditions. However, patients and providers should be aware that these conditions can be alleviated over time and that it's important to continue to evaluate the need for these medications, especially in older adults.

Antiseizure or Anticonvulsants

Antiseizure medications are used to reduce seizure activity. Some of these medications are also used as mood stabilizers in people with bipolar disorder and for nerve pain, also called neuropathy.

Antiseizure	
Hydantoin	phenytoin
Miscellaneous	carbamazepine, lamotrigine, levetiracetam, oxcarbazepine, topiramate, valproic acid, zonisamide

Information on when and how to reduce or deprescribe antiseizure medications is minimal at best. I have personally counseled patients in their 70s who had been taking antiseizure medicines since they had a seizure when they were in their 20s, although they had never experienced another episode. Antiseizure medications are prescribed to reduce the risk of seizure relapse, and a patient who has experienced seizures may be apprehensive about reducing or stopping such medications. This is especially true for those who drive and do not want to have a seizure while driving or be forced to stop driving as a temporary precaution if the medication is changed.

But seizure medications can lead to osteoporosis, fatigue, hair loss, liver toxicity, skin reactions, and hematological changes. The article "Deprescribing in Epilepsy: Do No Harm"[46] highlights the difficulty in deprescribing these medications and the importance of risk assessment and patient preference in the process. As you can imagine, many variables, including type of seizure and time elapsed since the last seizure, affect the ability to deprescribe these types of medication.

Benzodiazepines

Benzodiazepines are medications used to reduce anxiety and enhance sleep. They tend to be used episodically and on an as-needed basis when someone may be suffering from insomnia or feeling anxious.

Benzodiazepines
alprazolam, clonazepam, diazepam, lorazepam, oxazepam, temazepam, triazolam

Benzodiazepines are best to be used only minimally and should be reduced and eventually deprescribed, as they can affect cognition and increase confusion and fall risk. If you suffer from chronic anxiety or have had multiple anxious episodes throughout the years, you should talk to your health-care provider about other types of medication that are more suited to long-term use rather than taking a benzodiazepine for each episode. Think about it: reducing the occurrence of anxiety/panic episodes may in itself make you feel better. Other medications for chronic anxiety include some of the ones highlighted in the antidepressant category, including the SSRIs sertraline and citalopram, for example.

Years ago, when I was working in a retail pharmacy, a daughter of an older adult customer came to the pharmacy to pick up her mother's prescriptions. She mentioned that her mother had fallen multiple times. Reviewing the woman's medications, I warned that the diazepam her mother was taking could be increasing her risk of falls. Older adults' bodies can take longer to eliminate diazepam, a long-acting benzodiazepine, resulting in a build-up of the medication. I suggested that they should review the prescription with her mother's doctor and ask about reducing the medication or changing it to a shorter-acting benzodiazepine such as lorazepam to begin the tapering process. The daughter replied, "You will never get those away from her."

I was a bit surprised at the response, although I had seen similar reactions in other patients. People become attached to particular medications, especially if they have been used for years for acute anxious situations.

Months passed before I saw the daughter again. She caught my attention to tell me she had found a new doctor for her mother, a geriatrician, and that I was right: the new doctor had quickly deprescribed the diazepam and her mother was no longer falling. This anecdote illustrates the education, resistance, time, and effort it can take to deprescribe, especially when preconceived notions of medication attachment and reluctance to stop are barriers to change.

A Closer Look: Benzodiazepines

A 2014 study, "Eliminating Medications through Patient Ownership of End Results (EMPOWER),"[47] provides compelling evidence that educating patients can help reduce polypharmacy and facilitate shared decision-making with prescribers and pharmacists alike. In this study, health-care consumers were provided an educational pamphlet regarding the risks of benzodiazepines. An overwhelming majority of patients were pleased to receive the information, and many tried to act on it.

The study showed that all of the participants who stopped taking the benzodiazepine benefitted and suffered no adverse reaction to the discontinuation. Positive results were noted for men and women, over and under 80 years of age, and of varying education and health levels. Diagnosis, dose, number of other prescriptions, or a previous attempt to stop a benzodiazepine did not affect these positive results.

However, the study also revealed that education of health-care providers is required for successful and sound deprescribing, as not all study participants received a positive response when they approached their providers with the information they had learned.

Some prescribers or pharmacists discouraged participants from reducing the benzodiazepine medication,
essentially telling the consumers that they should "wait
and see" if they developed negative side effects before
they would consider deprescribing the benzodiazepine.
Patients and physicians were also concerned about
withdrawal symptoms, even though a taper dosing
was suggested in the educational material. And some
patients were switched to medications that also posed
risk factors, especially in older adults.

Unfortunately, there is no one-size-fits-all to deprescribing. It is truly an individualized process with your
health-care providers. Good things take effort, even
deprescribing and optimizing your medications.

Bisphosphonates

Bisphosphonates are used to build bone and improve bone density.
They are regularly prescribed to offset the effects of osteoporosis or
bone cancer.

Bisphosphonates
alendronate, ibandronate, risedronate

Sometimes medications are continued beyond the time in which
even the medication's own guidelines would say it should be stopped,
as is the case with bisphosphonates, which have a timeline of use.
The first evaluation to consider, whether these medications should be
continued, is at the three-to-five-year mark. If your bone density has
not increased enough at that point and/or you are still at high risk for
a fracture, then the medication may be continued for up to 10 years,
maximum. Beyond 10 years, bisphosphonates are not therapeutically

helpful and cause more side effects, such as stomach and esophagus ulcers, difficulty swallowing, heartburn, and muscle and bone pain.

I talk to many patients who cannot remember how long they have been taking this type of medication. I try to help by asking, "More than three years? More than five years? Do you think it has been ten years?" My next question is, "When was your last bone mineral density scan?" I think it's a bad sign when the patients cannot recall how long they have been taking the medication or when they last had a bone density scan. I explain the time limit of this medicine and suggest they check with their doctor to schedule a bone density scan to determine if they should continue the prescription.

Bisphosphonates should not be taken for more than ten years, even if patients take a break from the medication for a few years. The clock does not start over with each reintroduction of the drug; it's the total number of years that matters.

Blood Pressure Medications

Blood pressure medications are also called antihypertensives. There are many categories of this type of medication, which are used to reduce blood pressure and typically need to be taken indefinitely for continued blood pressure control.

Blood Pressure Medications	
ACE inhibitors	benazepril, captopril, enalapril, lisinopril, quinapril
ARBs	losartan, olmesartan, valsartan
Beta-blockers	atenolol, metoprolol, nebivolol
Calcium channel blockers	amlodipine, diltiazem, verapamil
Diuretics: Loop	bumetanide, ethacrynic acid, furosemide, torsemide
Potassium-sparing	amiloride, eplerenone, spironolactone, triamterene
Thiazide	chlorthalidone, hydrochlorothiazide

Blood pressure medications can be beneficial in reducing progression of heart disease, heart attacks, strokes, and the risk of kidney disease. Multiple medications may be necessary to lower blood pressure; however, those medications need to be reduced or removed as people age. Blood pressure goals can also vary and become less stringent with age, health status, and patient sensitivity to side effects.

Some blood pressure medications, such as diuretics, can cause lightheadedness, dizziness, low blood pressure, decreased heart rate, dehydration, or electrolyte imbalance, all of which increase the risk of falls, injury, or other cardiovascular events. Such symptoms may call for a reduction in the medication.

Calcium channel blockers can increase the risk of edema, causing swollen feet and ankles, a condition that is especially concerning in people who have heart failure. Adjusting blood pressure medications by reducing or stopping the calcium channel blocker may reduce the risk of heart failure exacerbation that can lead to hospitalizations.

Dementia Medications

Dementia medications help to slow the progression of cognitive deficits. There are many forms of dementia, with the most common being Alzheimer's disease.

Dementia Medications	
Acetylcholinesterase inhibitors	donepezil, galantamine, rivastigmine
NMDA receptor antagonist	memantine

These medications can be one of the most difficult groups of medications to deprescribe, and it is estimated that a third of dementia medications are unnecessarily continued. Dementia medications are tricky. Not everyone responds to them, and they can trigger several side effects. And the medications often have no therapeutic benefit after a time, even for people who were helped by them initially.

Common dementia medications, such as donepezil, can cause urinary incontinence or overactive bladder, and this side effect is frequently treated with a medication such as oxybutynin, which counteracts the effectiveness of the donepezil. The oxybutynin may be helpful to reduce the urinary incontinence, but it may interfere with donepezil, negating any positive cognitive effects, and it also increases the risk of falls.

As mentioned in an interview with Dr. Emily Reeve, health-care providers should discuss the prospect of deprescribing dementia medications at the time the medicines are initially prescribed.[48] If a person is taking medications for dementia and benefitting without side effects, then by all means continue the medication. However, the use of the drugs should be reevaluated every six months, and caregivers and health-care providers should regularly look for signs of a prescribing cascade or worsening of the patient's dementia. If the patient's dementia is worsening or if new medications are being added to counteract side effects of the dementia drugs, it may be time to deprescribe the dementia drugs. Of course, this may be a difficult decision for the individual, family, and caregivers.

It is best to taper dementia medications slowly. Monitoring is most important to gauge worsening of dementia or withdrawal symptoms such as hallucinations, anxiety, agitation, and altered mental status.

Diabetes Medications

Diabetes medications help reduce blood glucose by moving glucose from the blood into the cells to produce energy. Many medications are used to treat type 2 diabetes. Insulin is the only medication that can be used for type 1 diabetes.

Diabetes Medications	
Biguanide	metformin
DDP-4 inhibitors	linagliptin, saxagliptin, sitagliptin
Insulin	insulin-aspart, -degludec, -detemir, -glargine, -lispro, -NPH, -regular
Meglitinide	nateglinide, repaglinide
SGLT2 inhibitor	canagliflozin, dapagliflozin, empagliflozin
Sulfonylureas	glipizide, glyburide, glimepiride
Thiazolidinedione	pioglitazone, rosiglitazone

There are two types of diabetes: type 1 and type 2. Type 1 diabetes means the body is not making insulin; therefore, the only treatment is insulin. Type 2 diabetes is more complex in that insulin is made but not used efficiently by the body; therefore, other medications are needed to support the use of insulin, produce more insulin, or reduce glucose release and availability. Type 2 diabetes can progress to the point of requiring insulin use, but it can also be reversed through lifestyle changes, including reducing weight; balancing nutrition of carbohydrates, fats, and proteins; and increasing activity levels.

When treating either type of diabetes, it is important to be aware of hypoglycemia, or low blood sugar, which can cause you to feel shaky, confused, or moody and increase your heart rate. Sugar is needed immediately to treat a hypoglycemic episode, and you can get it by taking glucose tablets, hard candy, honey, juice, or soda. Hypoglycemia can quickly cause a person to lose consciousness, which can increase falls and require a trip to the emergency department. As they age, people taking medications for diabetes may become more susceptible to hypoglycemic episodes and may have reduced awareness of warning signs. Or patients may need less medication over time if they lose weight or have other changes in their body.

Diabetes is commonly treated with multiple medications. If you are diagnosed with type 2 diabetes in your 50s, you may be prescribed several medications to treat your diabetes as you age. But what happens when you retire and have time to change your lifestyle? You may start to walk more and eat healthier. You may become more active now than you were when you used to commute for hours and then spend the day at your desk, and you are not as likely stopping for fast food or eating out for multiple lunch meetings. Such lifestyle changes can mean that older adults may no longer need all of their prescribed diabetes medications, because their HbA1c (blood test to determine average blood glucose) levels have decreased to an appropriate range.

Certain medications are also more likely to cause hypoglycemic episodes, especially in older adults. The family of sulfonylureas, which include glyburide and glipizide, are commonly known to cause an increased risk of low blood sugar. The risk is so well-known that some insurances have added prior authorizations or decided to no longer cover these medications as a safety precaution. If you are experiencing low blood sugar levels, adjustments may need to be made to your medications. Though low blood sugar can be treated with sugar, these episodes should be avoided due to the risk of consequences such as falls and arrhythmias.

A newer family of medication for diabetes, known as "flozins," increases the elimination of glucose through the kidneys and urine. This type of medication can be very helpful; however, it can also lead to an increase in urinary tract infections (UTIs) due to the increased glucose in the urine. And UTIs can frequently cause confusion and altered mental status for older adults.

In one example, a patient came to the hospital due to a hypoglycemic episode and a UTI— the second one the patient had experienced since beginning this new type of diabetes medication. On top of that, a review of the patient's HbA1c levels revealed that they were well within range to deprescribe the medication and to monitor the patient. The patient's providers decided to stop the flozin.

The second issue regarding this case was that the patient was also taking a once-daily dose of long-acting insulin. When adding oral diabetes medications for patients who are using insulin, it is recommended that the insulin dose be reduced during initiation of the new agent, to prevent hypoglycemia.

Diphenhydramine

Diphenhydramine and other over-the-counter (OTC) antihistamines—especially the first-generation products (the ones that have been around for years)—are used in medicines to alleviate allergies and also in sleep aids and night-time cough and cold medicines.

Antihistamines	
First Generation	brompheniramine, chlorpheniramine, clemastine, diphenhydramine, doxylamine, meclizine
Second Generation	cetirizine, fexofenadine, loratadine

OTC products, including pain relief medicines, "PM" or other nighttime products, antihistamines, cough and cold products, and sleep aids typically contain an active ingredient called diphenhydramine (pronounced di-fen-hi-dra-mean.) Diphenhydramine can cause a multitude of side effects, especially in older adults, and it lasts many hours longer in their bodies than it does in younger adults. Side effects include dry eyes, dry mouth, and difficulty urinating. It can also cause sleepiness (hence the reason it is used in nighttime products), but this sleepiness can last longer in older adults, resulting in an effect that many people describe as a "hangover" the morning after taking a diphenhydramine product. Other side effects include slowed cognition, confusion, and increased heart rate, which can trigger possible arrhythmias and increase the risk of falls.

When I see diphenhydramine on a patient's list of medications, I always question the need. This is one medication that older adults should avoid. People who are having trouble sleeping should first try nonmedication actions, such as lifestyle changes, and give them time to work well. Reducing caffeine and avoiding chocolate after midafternoon is a good first step, as is being active and avoiding napping during the day. I have spoken with many people who fall asleep during the day and then wonder why they cannot sleep at night. Reducing stimulation and computer or phone lighting (known as blue light, which reduces the activation of circadian triggers for inducing sleep) in the evening and reading from a traditional book may also improve sleep.

I relayed this sleep information to a group of older adults who were at an outreach event to learn more about medications and falls and to participate in a medication review. When I explained that diphenhydramine is a high-risk medication that can increase falls, the participants all looked at each other, wide-eyed. Then one of the women said, "That must be what happened to Helen last night—she must have taken her 'pain PM' medication!" Helen had fallen in the middle of the night and been taken by ambulance to the emergency department.

Another woman called the outreach program because she was experiencing a reaction to an insect bite. The reaction was not life-threatening; however, she wanted advice as to what to do and what she could take. This woman, who was in her 80s, wanted to take diphenhydramine to help ease the reaction. Instead, I suggested loratadine, a newer antihistamine with milder side effects that appeared to be appropriate with her other medications. She had both products on hand but wanted to take the diphenhydramine. I explained that loratadine is a much safer product and would still help with the reaction she was experiencing. When I explained that the diphenhydramine could increase her risk of falls, she stated that her husband was present and would catch her. How wonderful that she trusted her husband so much! I stated again that loratadine is a better choice. She then said she would call her doctor, who she expected would approve the diphenhydramine!

A Closer Look: Medications that interfere with sleep

Problems getting to sleep or staying asleep can make many people want to reach for an OTC sleep medication. Making changes to your sleep patterns, diet, or lifestyle may help you reduce the need for sleep aids, which can have many harmful side effects, especially for older adults.

Bupropion, a medication for depression or smoking cessation, can interfere with sleep. Bupropion is best taken before midafternoon, especially if multiple doses are prescribed. Nicotine is also stimulating; therefore, if you use a patch to stop smoking, remove the patch before bedtime. If you have a craving for a cigarette first thing in the morning, use nicotine gum or a lozenge when you wake up and apply the patch at the same time. This will allow time for the patch to begin to work while you have also addressed the acute craving. If you take diuretics, take them earlier in the day, no later than midafternoon, if possible. Taking them too late in the evening can cause you to be up all night because you have to urinate.

Alcohol can make us sleepy initially, but it has an excitatory side effect a few hours later that may wake you up and make it hard to fall back to sleep. Chocolate and caffeine and can also keep you awake.

Eyedrops for Glaucoma

Few people realize that eyedrops can have effects on their whole body.

Eyedrops for Glaucoma	
Carbonic anhydrase inhibitors	brinzolamide, dorzolamide
Beta blocker	timolol
Prostaglandin analog	bimatoprost, latanoprost, travoprost

I remember one of the first times I explained the correct use of eyedrops at a program at a local older adult community center. Instill one drop in your eye and then either close your eye or hold your finger to the side of your eye by your nose to block off the tear duct for one minute. You should do this to allow the eyedrop to work in the eye while blocking the medicine from entering the tear duct, potentially causing quick, systemic side effects of the medicine that may affect the heart or lungs. The audience was astounded, and they wanted to know why no one had ever told them that before. I really did not have an answer but assured them that they could achieve better therapeutic outcomes if they administered their eyedrops in this manner. Drops should also be instilled one at a time with a few minutes in-between, as the eye can only hold one drop at a time. Multiple drops instilled without a pause will roll down the cheek as expensive tears.

Timolol, an eyedrop to fight glaucoma, should be used in this manner to reduce possible systemic effects. Timolol is a nonselective beta-blocker that may slow the heart rate or constrict the airways of the lungs. These effects can cause dizziness, chest discomfort, shortness of breath, and—you guessed it—falls.

Dorzolamide, another eyedrop used for glaucoma, needs to be eliminated from your system, as all medications do. It is not recommended for use in patients with severe kidney dysfunction, as it can cause toxicities and lead to anemia. There are safer alternatives. Ask your health-care provider about switching from a carbonic anhydrase inhibitor like dorzolamide to a different class of medication (such as a prostaglandin analog—for example, latanoprost).

Gabapentin

Gabapentin, originally approved for seizures, is typically used for neuropathic pain, including diabetic neuropathy, and nerve pain from shingles.

GABA analog
gabapentin, pregabalin

Some medications may need a change in dosing as well as frequency, depending upon a user's age, kidney function, and/or liver function. Gabapentin is one medication that needs to be dosed carefully, especially in older adults, as kidney function can negatively affect its elimination, increasing the risk of falls and side effects.

Gabapentin has quite a range of dosing, especially for nerve pain (neuropathy). Maximum daily doses for generally healthy adults with good working kidneys is 3,600 mg per 24 hours. Typically, this is taken in divided doses of 1,200 mg three times throughout the day. For someone on hemodialysis (a process that filters an individual's blood if one's kidneys are unhealthy and unable to do so), the dose drops to 300 mg three times per week. That's quite a significant difference in dosing!

There are several recommended ranges between these doses, mainly related to kidney function, but this illustrates the vast difference. If the medication is not reviewed, patients can easily continue to take gabapentin at high doses over the years, and these levels could eventually lead to problems. With diabetes, kidney function tends to decrease over time, and patients may end up in the emergency department with a fall or confusion if their prescribed dose of gabapentin remains too high.

Gabapentin can also become a problem if patients take OTC pain relievers, such as ibuprofen or naproxen for pain or fever. Most users think these OTC drugs are harmless, but these NSAIDs can also reduce kidney function, which can add to the problematic effects of gabapentin. Some patients may not even realize that there are NSAIDs in combination OTC products used for pain and headaches. Many of those types of products include both acetaminophen and an NSAID. At times we see acute changes in kidney function (also known as acute kidney injury) that will add to possible toxicity of medications like gabapentin.

For example, Mr. N lands in the hospital due to dizziness, orthostatic hypotension, vertigo, and gait issues. The patient has been taking gabapentin 200 mg three times a day, which is equal to 600 mg daily or 4200 mg per week. Due to poor kidney function, the patient is on hemodialysis; therefore, the dosing should be 300 mg three times per week, for a total of 900 mg per week. That is a big difference in dosing! Gabapentin toxicity can result in dizziness, orthostatic hypotension, and gait issues, as seen by Mr. N. Reducing the dose of gabapentin to 300 mg three times per week, on hemodialysis days, will still offer Mr. N relief from neuropathic pain but should reduce falls, confusion, and toxicity from the medication.

Herbals

I have had some interesting encounters with patients who take herbals. What surprises me most is the number of herbals some patients take—even though they are not sure why they are taking them or the expected purpose of each one. Many individuals think that because herbals are natural, they must be safe. This just is not true. Too much of some herbals or incorrect combinations can have detrimental effects.

Some herbal formulas have effects on blood glucose, which could cause increased or decreased blood glucose and worsen diabetes or hypoglycemia, especially if combined with medications that can also cause hypoglycemia. Many products have hormonal effects, while others may increase or decrease blood pressure. These are important concerns as many people live with high blood pressure and diabetes.

One patient who had suffered a stroke wanted to have her medications reviewed. The patient was taking three combination herbal products, each containing several herbal ingredients (totaling 32 herbals!), as well as single products and supplements. Notably, neither single herbals nor combination products are approved or regulated by the FDA. Many herbals in the combined products could have increased her blood pressure, and another herbal had side effects of increased estrogen, which could increase the risk of clotting. She was using the combination as an attempt to ease the effects of hormonal changes due to menopause, but it may have increased her blood pressure and the risk of blood clots, thereby increasing the risk of stroke. Especially concerning were the underlying conditions of high blood pressure and increased cardiovascular risk for postmenopausal women.

Iron Supplements

Iron supplements are frequently continued beyond the time when they are truly needed. An unfortunate side effect of iron is constipation. The patient then self-treats or is instructed to take laxatives and stool softeners, leading to a classic example of a prescribing cascade, where one medication is started and another is added due to a side effect of the first medication. In cases like this, people may take medications to combat the discomfort of constipation when the iron could be reduced or stopped, which could relieve the constipation and the need for other medications.

Nonsteroidal Anti-Inflammatory Drugs (NSAIDs)

NSAIDs can be found in OTC or prescription products that help alleviate pain, inflammation, and fever. NSAIDs are available in prescription strength, prescription medication combinations, and widely available in both single and combination OTC products.

NSAIDs
diclofenac, ibuprofen, naproxen, meloxicam

People reach for OTC pain relief for sore muscles, back pain, headaches, knee pain, or general aches. These can be obtained at the grocery store, gas station, or pharmacy, and from family and friends. NSAIDs, including ibuprofen, naproxen, and aspirin, for example, are marketed under various brand names and are included in combination medications such as pain relief for migraines and cough and cold and allergy medications.

And because many of these are sold without prescriptions, we think they are safe for anyone to take. This is far from true, and many people wind up in the hospital every year because of problems caused or worsened by NSAIDs. People with kidney disease, heart failure, or hypertension especially need to be aware that NSAIDs can make their conditions worse.

IN REAL LIFE

Here are a few scenarios involving NSAIDs that bring people to the emergency department.

Mr. A, an older man with heart failure, is experiencing shortness of breath, ankle edema, and has difficulty urinating. He has recently been taking ibuprofen for knee pain. Ibuprofen in his case has caused a worsening kidney function and exacerbation of heart failure. Mr. A was admitted to the hospital for diuresis protocol.

Mrs. B, who takes common blood pressure medication such as lisinopril or losartan and a diuretic, reaches for naproxen whenever she experiences back pain. Though she may currently have normal kidney function, an interaction between the blood pressure medication, diuretic, and NSAID can cause an acute kidney injury, which can land a patient in the hospital. These very common medications should not be combined. If pain management is needed by someone on these meds, acetaminophen is typically the safer option.

Ms. C, who has been taking the maximum dosing of citalopram for her anxiety, grabbed an ibuprofen instead of her typical acetaminophen when she had a headache, not knowing that combining SSRIs used for depression or anxiety and an NSAID can increase chances for stomach bleed. She had to be hospitalized and treated for a GI bleed. Other OTC products, such as omega-3 and garlic, act as blood-thinning aids. When many of these products are combined, the risk of a bleed increases.

Proton Pump Inhibitors (PPIs)

Proton pump inhibitors reduce the acid in the stomach to help alleviate acid reflux, heartburn, and ulcers.

Proton Pump Inhibitors (PPIs)
dexlansoprazole, esomeprazole, lansoprazole, omeprazole, pantoprazole, rabeprazole

Over the past few decades, long-term use of PPIs has become a far too common way to treat gastroesophageal reflux disease (GERD), also known as gastric reflux or acid reflux. PPIs should be used only for a short period of time, approximately two weeks, to resolve this acute condition. Many people, however, have remained on these medications for years.

There are many uses for PPIs including prophylactically in the hospital to prevent ulcers or to prevent a stomach or gastro-intestinal

(GI) bleed for people on blood thinners. PPIs may also be prescribed for more significant gastric acid conditions such as Barrett's esophagus. However, if chronic conditions do not exist, then the PPI is not needed indefinitely.

Why is it important to stop a PPI if it is not needed? PPIs increase the pH of the stomach, making it less acidic. This increased pH interrupts the absorption of many nutrients that need a more acidic environment. These nutrients include vitamin B12, vitamin D, magnesium, calcium, and iron, and all play an important role in your general well-being.

Vitamin B12 is important for balance, brain activity, and nerve health. Deficiency of vitamin B12 may cause tingling of the hands and feet, memory loss, anemia, and difficulty with balance. Vitamin D is important for muscle and bone health and helps with the absorption of calcium. Deficiency in vitamin D can lead to weak bones and muscles and muscle aches. Magnesium is important for muscle function, including the heart. Anyone who has been on a PPI for a year or more should have a magnesium level check because low magnesium can cause arrythmias. Iron helps transport oxygen throughout our body and is commonly combined with vitamin C in some OTC products because vitamin C is an acid (ascorbic acid) that assists with the absorption of iron.

PPIs are also linked to an increased risk of falls and fractures, excessive diarrhea due to *Clostridium difficile* (C. *diff.*), and pneumonia. The interruption of the gut flora balance due to the increased pH may increase the diarrhea and pneumonia risks.

But many people who try to stop PPIs abruptly experience acid rebound, making them believe they need to continue taking the PPI. Stopping a PPI abruptly, especially if you have been taking it daily for three months or more, will typically cause terrible stomach acid symptoms, leading one to believe that the medication is most definitely necessary. Instead, PPIs should be slowly tapered over time to avoid this discomfort.

I have encountered numerous patients who continued on PPIs unnecessarily because they had a bad experience when they tried to stop taking them. I say, "Let me guess. You stopped the PPI abruptly, were doubled over in pain (due to acid rebound), and extremely uncomfortable. You decided that you needed to continue the medication. Years go by and you are still on the medication." I am often met with, "Yes! How did you know?"

Instead of trying to abruptly stop a PPI, you should be given a plan to reduce the medication slowly. For example, the medication is reduced to half the daily dose, perhaps for a week. Each week, it is lowered again by half, until you are taking the lowest dose available daily. Next, you take the lowest dose PPI every other day for a week. If you have difficulty on the "off days," you can take an antacid if needed. Gradually, you increase the number of "off days" each week. Once you are comfortably off the medication, you can take the PPI on an as-needed basis.

If an acidic stomach is a problem, try nondrug solutions such as adjusting your diet and activities. Learn which foods to avoid and which foods to add and how timing of food intake, reclining, and exercise can affect you. Eating a smaller quantity of food or eating less acidic food such as citrus, tomatoes, or spicy food may help. Reducing caffeine and carbonated products can also reduce gastric reflux. Foods that may help include yogurt or other foods with active cultures. Do not eat close to bedtime, and wait a couple of hours after eating before you lie down. Exercise can also help maintain or improve gastric movement to reduce reflux.

Statins

Statins reduce total cholesterol, increase HDL (the "good" cholesterol), and decrease LDL (the "bad" cholesterol). Keeping cholesterol in check helps cardiovascular (heart) health.

Statins
atorvastatin, fluvastatin, lovastatin, pitavastatin, pravastatin, rosuvastatin, simvastatin

The idea of deprescribing statins has become a controversial topic. Some studies show stopping statins may cause an increased risk of hospitalization and poor cardiovascular outcomes over time.[49, 50] Reviewing other studies with shorter time results, stopping the statin for 60 days, showed to be acceptable, while stopping a statin for two years time showed to be more problematic.[51] Older adults may benefit from continuing statins because cardiovascular risks increase with age; however, many studies on this issue do not have data for people older than 75 years to show whether the benefits outweigh the risks. Deprescribing statins should be individualized, with patient and provider considering adverse side effects, drug interactions, and life expectancy while determining the appropriateness of continuing the medication.

Statins have been shown to potentially cause muscle weakness over time in aging adults.[52] The weakness may occur so gradually that users may not realize that a medication could be causing the problem. But any medication that may contribute to muscle weakness could lead to reduced exercise and eventually falls. If someone is experiencing such problems, it could be time to consider reducing the statin to a lower dose and reevaluating cholesterol levels, muscle strength, and pain/discomfort.

A case of switching statins

Several years ago, Mr. R called the pharmacy outreach program and asked for a review of his medications, which included rosuvastatin (a statin), ezetimibe (to lower LDL cholesterol), niacin (to increase HDL cholesterol), lisinopril (for blood pressure), aspirin (for heart protection), and a PPI (for gastric acid reflux). Mr. R explained that he had been taking atorvastatin for some time prior to rosuvastatin, as rosuvastatin was not a generic at the time and atorvastatin was much less expensive. Unfortunately, atorvastatin was not as therapeutically effective for him, so ezetimibe was added to help reduce LDL and niacin was added to increase HDL. Eventually, rosuvastatin was available as a generic and was an affordable option, so the atorvastatin was changed to rosuvastatin. The ezetimibe and niacin were continued. He told me that the rosuvastatin was working very well and his cholesterol numbers were in check.

Now, you might think, "Great! Continue to take your medications since your cholesterol numbers are finally at an appropriate therapeutic outcome." I, on the other hand, said, "Wait! So you changed from atorvastatin to rosuvastatin and that is when your cholesterol numbers improved, but you have also continued on ezetimibe and niacin?" I suggested that since rosuvastatin had become the workhorse for the better cholesterol levels, the ezetimibe and niacin might not be needed. He was stunned and intrigued, particularly because he was finding the ezetimibe to be rather expensive. We formulated a plan for him to talk to his provider about deprescribing niacin and ezetimibe.

Feeling empowered and educated after our call, Mr. R discussed options with his prescriber, came up with a plan,

arrived at a decision, and went through the steps of deprescribing and monitoring. I consider this interaction a success
because many individuals who are interested in the education
and discussion never act or advocate for an actual change.

Conversations like the one I had with Mr. R make me
wonder how many people continue unnecessary medications.
In this man's case, half of his medications were unnecessary:
because one medication had changed, two others were no longer
necessary (and as a bonus the PPI that had been continued
needlessly was also deprescribed).

Supplements

Supplements support various body functions and can be helpful if
your body is lacking a particular vitamin, mineral, or other nutrient.
There are too many to list, but be certain to record any supplements
you take on your MedStrong Medication List.

Some supplements may interfere with lab tests and prevent an
accurate diagnosis. One patient had been admitted to a hospital more
than once for high calcium levels, which can be caused by problems
with the parathyroid, which regulates calcium, so measuring the
parathyroid hormone (PTH) is a key step in diagnosis. If PTH is
high, then hyperparathyroidism can be diagnosed as the culprit of
the high calcium levels. However, biotin, a supplement used for hair
and nail beauty, can interfere with the test and cause PTH levels to
falsely register as lower than they really are. When reviewing this
patient's medications, we learned she faithfully took high-dose biotin
two times daily and was so pleased because her hair and nails looked
great. In order for the patient to have a truly accurate PTH test, she
needed to stop biotin for three days, but she was discharged from
the hospital before the retest could be done. Educating the patient

and communicating about her need to follow up with her primary care provider became an important step.

Biotin can also interfere with cardiovascular enzymes when determining if someone is having a heart attack, as troponin levels may appear falsely low instead of elevated. Because biotin is an OTC, some patients fail to record it on their medication list. Be certain to let your providers know if you take biotin when you are having blood work.

Tramadol

Tramadol is used for acute or chronic pain management. It is part of the opioid family and used for moderate to moderately severe pain. Opioids will be reviewed further in chapter 8, but tramadol is being discussed here because it is often believed to be a better option to treat pain in older adults. However, that is not always true.

Opioids
oxycodone, hydrocodone, morphine, tramadol

I was asked to review the medications of an older male by his daughter, who said her father was just not "bouncing back" to his normal self after a recent surgery. She stated he was typically a very bright man—he had worked as a scientist for many years—who did not have dementia. When I reviewed his medications, I noticed that tramadol was being prescribed four weeks post-surgery. He had not been on this medication previously. In discussing this medication with the daughter, I learned she was not quite certain if the medication was helping with pain or if her dad even had pain any longer. We decided she would work with the doctor to taper the tramadol and eventually deprescribe the med. When we spoke a couple of weeks later, she told me her father was off the tramadol, back to his bright self, and not experiencing pain, and she thanked me for helping her and her father.

Caregivers tend to be hesitant to remove pain relievers, especially if they don't know whether the pain will return once the medication is stopped. But tramadol was having substantial effects on this individual, causing a geriatric syndrome of cognitive deficits, which could have been overlooked or never connected to the medication. The primary care physician may not have wanted to touch this medication, especially if a specialist prescribed it in the first place. A full month's supply had been provided at hospital discharge, and therefore the patient continued to take it for weeks instead of evaluating, after a shorter time, whether pain relief was truly necessary.

Other Surprises You Might Find in Your Pillbox

A careful examination of your pillbox may turn up drugs that interact badly with each other or prescriptions that exceed the maximum dosing for your age. Here are some examples of problems you might find.

Drug-drug interactions

Medications become riskier the older we become and the more we take. This direct correlation between drug-drug interaction, age, and number of medications tends to increase, and can build on each other. As noted previously, polypharmacy is also a global concern. One study that looked at these parameters found that two-thirds of patients 60 years and older had at least one drug-drug interaction amongst their medications. Those who were 70 years and older were even more likely to have one or multiple drug interactions with their medications.[53]

Drug-disease interactions

Drug-disease interactions are an important factor in the risk-versus-benefit paradigm of medications.[54] I'm listing just some of the more common drug-disease interactions here.

- Heart failure can worsen with NSAID use; however, people with heart failure are frequently unaware of this interaction.

- Calcium channel blockers (CCBs), a type of blood pressure medication that includes amlodipine, verapamil, and diltiazem, can cause edema, or water retention, and can lead to worsening or exacerbation of heart failure.

- Diabetes medications such as pioglitazone and rosiglitazone (TZDs) should not be used by patients with type 2 diabetes and heart failure, as they can cause fluid retention that can worsen heart failure.

- Dementia can be made worse by anticholinergics, benzodiazepines, antipsychotics, and sleep aids.

- NSAIDs can worsen kidney function even in people with normal kidney function, and should be avoided in people with reduced kidney function or chronic kidney disease. NSAIDs cause retention of water and sodium, causing edema, and can increase blood pressure.

- Decongestants can increase blood pressure and cause a fast heartbeat, potentially worsening high blood pressure and triggering arrhythmias.

- Nonselective beta-blockers can worsen conditions that cause breathing difficulty, such as COPD and asthma.

IN REAL LIFE

Drug-Disease Interactions

Mr. M has COPD and experiences anxiety, which is very common for those with COPD and asthma. Not being able to breathe will definitely make one anxious, and the opposite is also true: anxiety or a panic episode can cause shortness of breath. Along with anxiety, patients may also experience rapid heart rate. Mr. M was prescribed a long-acting inhaler to control his COPD, a short-acting rescue inhaler for episodes of shortness of breath, and a nebulizer for added treatment when necessary. He was also prescribed propranolol for increased heart rate and sertraline for anxiety. Propranolol is a nonselective beta-blocker, which means it can reduce heart rate but also acts on other beta receptors found in the lungs that can cause airway restriction. A more selective beta-blocker for the heart receptors, such as metoprolol, to slow Mr. M's heart rate without affecting his lungs, might be a better option in this case.

This scenario illustrates a need to treat both increased heart rate and COPD with the safest options available for a patient with challenging health conditions. Part of the deprescribing process is to switch to medications that reduce the risk of drug-disease interactions. It is certainly important to reduce the heart rate but just as important to limit potential side effects and possible exacerbation of a COPD episode, which may lead to more anxiety, an unwelcome vicious cycle.

Your body is interconnected, medications have many effects, and treatment can be challenging. Keep the possibility of drug-disease interactions in mind when you are reviewing your medications and consider the following two points:

- Older medications may worsen new-found health conditions.

- Newer medications may worsen previously discovered health conditions.

～

Maximum dosing problems

Medication dosing may need to change due to kidney function, age, or other factors, but the dosage should not be increased without good reason and documentation. Some patients think, "If one is good, two must be better!" We have seen poor outcomes based on this impulse with antidepressants, aspirin, and supplements. Unfortunately, increasing medications may increase the risk of adverse drug reactions or side effects. The other caution is that what should be the maximum dose of particular medications can change as we age. Here are some examples of what can happen with some common medications.

Citalopram. Maximum dosing for citalopram, an antidepressant/antianxiety medication, for adults is 40 mg once daily; however, 20 mg once daily is the maximum for those age 65 years and older. Does this mean that if you are taking citalopram 40 mg it needs to be lowered to 20 mg on your 65th birthday? Probably not; however, it should be reviewed and possibly tapered down over time. If you are 80 years old and still taking citalopram 40 mg, a reduction in dose is most likely warranted, especially if you are experiencing cardiovascular changes.

For example, an older adult was brought to the hospital for cardiovascular issues; it was found on her tests for heart rhythm that the QT interval—a segment of the heart wave you may have seen on television shows or advertisements or watching a heart monitor—was prolonged. When her medication list was reviewed, there were medications that may have had an additive effect on this type of heart-beat irregularity, and one in particular stood out. She was taking citalopram 20 mg two times daily. Typically, citalopram is dosed once-daily. Reducing her dose to citalopram 20 mg daily allowed for a favorable dosing of the medication for her age and decreased the QT interval to a normal interval.

Simvastatin. Maximum dosing problems may arise due to the combination of medications. A common example is amlodipine used for blood pressure and simvastatin used for cholesterol. Amlodipine can increase simvastatin availability, which can cause increased side effects, such as muscle aches and weakness. The maximum dose of simvastatin when combined with amlodipine should be 20 mg.

For example, a 91-year-old patient was taking amlodipine 10 mg and simvastatin 80 mg. When the patient complained of muscle aches and pains, the simvastatin dose was lowered to the 20 mg maximum, and the symptoms improved.

Zolpidem. A common prescription medication used for sleep, zolpidem, is dosed less in females than in males due to an increased time needed to eliminate the dose in females. The recommended dose of zolpidem is 5 mg for females versus 10 mg for males, to be taken at bedtime. But for older adults, the maximum dose is 5 mg, regardless of the patient's gender. Zolpidem can increase the risk of falls and, according to the Beer's Criteria, is a medication to avoid in older adults. When I see patients who say they have had multiple falls and are taking zolpidem, I check to make sure it is at the 5 mg dose. The next step is to have the patient and prescriber work together to slowly reduce the dose, especially if the medication has been taken for an extended period of time.

Educated, Enlightened, Empowered

This chapter has touched on a plethora of information and thrown around a lot of tongue-twister names that may not be familiar to anyone who is not working in the health-care industry. But it hopefully has enlightened you and illustrated to patients and health-care providers alike that many familiar medications can cause problems and that the risk-benefit analysis differs from person to person.

Use what you have learned here and keep reviewing your medications with all your health-care providers to optimize your medications and your health outcomes. Remember that deprescribing can be a beneficial treatment option that can make you feel and function better and may even alleviate a geriatric syndrome that concerns you or, better yet, avoid one all together!

In the next chapter, we will explore more potential concerns that can occur and also see that not all changes are necessarily correct and appropriate.

Wait....What? Just like any other change or nonchange, medications need to be constantly reviewed. Remember that Step 5 of the MedStrong Medication Optimization Plan (MOP) requires monitoring, documentation, and follow-up. Embrace that deprescribing is a constant consideration just like health checks, lifestyle changes, and taking helpful medications appropriately. If you "DO," you will be empowered to take a more active role in maintaining your health.

CHAPTER 8

Pitfalls and TrainRx

SETBACKS HAPPEN THROUGHOUT OUR LIFETIME, but health setbacks can truly impact quality of life and be especially challenging for an older adult. Some setbacks can be prevented though, if we learn what dangers to avoid. Falls and multiple hospitalizations can be hazardous to your health, so it's important to take proactive steps to avoid those pitfalls.

You've already read many times in this book that inappropriate medications or combinations of medications can increase your fall risk, but this issue is so important that it will be addressed in more depth in this chapter. We will pay particular attention to which medications should not be combined and look at a situation that can be especially tricky to navigate: transitions of care.

More knowledge. More empowerment. Better ability to complete Step 5 of the MedStrong Medication Optimization Plan (MOP): monitor, document, follow up.

Hazardous Medication Combinations

When we consider medications that should never be placed on the same drug list, we have to start by looking at opioids, which have been mentioned but not examined in depth up to this point. Opioids are used for pain management and can be used for acute pain and chronic pain; however, they should be reserved for severe pain situations where nonsteroidal anti-inflammatory drugs (NSAIDs) and acetaminophen are not effective.

Opioids pose a great risk to older adults, as they can cause falls, confusion, and constipation. Too often, medications are then prescribed to reduce the side effects, resulting in polypharmacy.

Opioids need to be prescribed judiciously, as we have learned from the recent opioid epidemic. And it's even more important that health-care providers review all of a patient's medications before adding opioids, as some medications need an extra layer of care and diligence, including the ones listed here.

Benzodiazepines, muscle relaxants, and opioids. These medications can cause respiratory depression and are linked to overdose—both intentional and unintentional.

Benzodiazepines and opioids. These two together can pose problems, including respiratory depression and overdose potential. Adding alcohol to these medications further increases their risks and the potential for overdose. The combination can increase the risk of death.

Gabapentin and opioids. Gabapentin is typically used for neuropathy or nerve pain and commonly prescribed for people who experience diabetic neuropathy or who have prolonged neuropathy after shingles. Opioids tend to be used for nociceptive pain, which occurs after surgery or traumatic injury, due to damage to tissue or bone. When both types of pain are present, nerve and nociceptive, both an opioid and gabapentin may be prescribed, especially if an individual who has been taking gabapentin for years experiences an injury or a surgery that results in an opioid prescription. These medications together can increase the risk of overdose by causing severe breathing difficulties.[56] The higher the dose, the higher the risk of death from a combination of gabapentin and opioids.[57] The combination not only increases gabapentin levels in the body, but also increases how the body is affected by gabapentin, enhancing side effects.

Multiple medications that affect the central nervous system. Health-care providers are increasingly prescribing medications such as opioids, benzodiazepines / tranquilizers, antidepressants, and antipsychotics separately and in combination for older adults.[58] This polypharmacy of sorts can have concerning impact on falls, driving, memory, and cognition. These medications are at times continued and used even without a formal diagnosis of depression, anxiety, insomnia, or pain.

Transitions of Care

Polypharmacy becomes particularly problematic during transitions of care, such as when someone moves from a hospital to a rehab facility or from one skilled nursing setting to another. Facilities and pharmacies may use different generics or brands, so you or the person you care for could end up with more than one version of the same medicine on your medication list. Medications may also be changed based on facility formularies.

As you can imagine, medication reconciliation is an important step when someone moves from one place to another. The medication list should be checked closely during a transition to make sure all medications are necessary, none have been duplicated, and no medicines have been added or deleted inadvertently.

IN REAL LIFE

What happened to Mrs. L illustrates the perils that can occur during care transitions.

Mrs. L was hospitalized for osteoarthritis knee surgery and was moving to a skilled nursing facility to complete her recovery. Because her blood pressure was rather low, her medications were reviewed and it was discovered that she was taking two similar blood pressure medications: lisinopril and losartan. Because these are similar classes of medications, they are typically not to be taken together.

When Mrs. L was asked if she was indeed taking both medications, she confirmed that she regularly took both. When asked if one medication had ever been prescribed to replace the other, she was uncertain. As Mrs. L's hospital pharmacy team looked further into the matter, it was discovered that she had been on both medications for almost a year and experienced several falls during that time, which could have been caused by low blood pressure and orthostatic hypotension.

It was further noted that auto-refills were occurring for both medications. It was then confirmed that the primary care physician had intended for Mrs. L to stop lisinopril and switch to losartan, not to add a new medication. The physician gladly called the skilled nursing facility to change the medication appropriately.

Mrs. L's story shows how medications can perpetuate unintentionally. That's why it is important for patient medications to be reviewed regularly, at the doctor's office, with the specialist, at the hospital, and at the pharmacy.

Double-checking "old" and "new" medications after a hospital stay or any change of care setting is an important step to prevent duplication of therapy, such as the same medication that may be prescribed in different formulations that are dosed differently. Let's look at metoprolol tartrate and metoprolol succinate, for example. Both can be prescribed for heart rate and high blood pressure, but the tartrate form is taken two times a day and the succinate is an extended release taken once daily. Or consider isosorbide dinitrate and isosorbide mononitrate, both of which widen blood vessels and can be used to prevent chest pain. The dinitrate formula is dosed two times daily and the mononitrate is dosed one time daily. Some facilities may have only one form available for their patients—even if the patient has been taking the other version. There certainly can be confusion if someone leaves a hospital or skilled nursing facility with a prescription for metoprolol tartrate, which they begin to take along with the metoprolol succinate they were taking previously. Problems also arise if a patient who was taking the once-daily dose at home but was given the twice-daily medication in the hospital returns home and starts taking his once-a-day dose twice a day—inadvertently doubling the dose.

Let's look at how some of these problems can play out for patients.

Ms. D, who had been prescribed isosorbide dinitrate and isosorbide mononitrate, was admitted to the hospital due to a fall. Isosorbide which can cause orthostatic hypotension, a drop in blood pressure when changing positions, which can cause lightheadedness, dizziness, and fainting. The medication also can cause a low heart rate. Taking both can, of course, have an additive effect. It is therefore not surprising that Ms. D experienced a fall due to the duplication of medication. At discharge, the hospitalist noted the duplication and gave specific instructions to the patient to stop taking the isosorbide dinitrate and take only the isosorbide mononitrate.

Mr. S experienced a problem that can occur with two medications that are commonly used to treat type 2 diabetes: glipizide and glyburide. These medications are very similar and are often substituted, one for the other, due to formularies and availability at facilities and with insurance companies. But during transitions of care, these two medications can be easily added or switched, and both can cause hypoglycemia, or low blood sugar. When Mr. S was hospitalized, his medication was switched from glyburide to glipizide at the hospital, due to the hospital formulary. When he returned to his long-term care facility, glipizide was added instead of being switched with glyburide. It wasn't long before Mr. S returned to the hospital due to hypoglycemia.

When Mrs. V went the hospital, she took medications for seizure control that were not on the hospital formulary. During her hospital stay, her seizure medication was changed to the hospital's formulary medication. Mrs. V was discharged with a prescription for the new anti-seizure medication, but she returned home and mistakenly began taking both medications. She soon had to return to the hospital for cardiovascular side effects caused by the combination of the two medications.

Medication Therapy Management (MTM)

Medication Therapy Management (MTM) is a means to review your medications at least on a yearly basis, if not more frequently, and is especially important after transitions of care have occurred. MTM is offered by insurance companies, especially those contracted with Medicare, and is a means of empowering the patient/caregiver to be the best advocate. The process helps patients ask questions and have the time to review the need, dose, frequency, interactions, and side effects of each medication. Unfortunately, not everyone can qualify for an MTM. We will be taking a closer look at this inconsistency in Part III of the book.

Using the MedStrong Medication Optimization Plan (MOP) from this book can be helpful whether or not you have access to MTM.

The Pitfall of Falls: A Good Reason to Deprescribe!

Falls are typically a culmination of many factors, including environment, medications, health conditions, and sensory impairment, and most individuals face more risks as they age. Each factor poses unique risks, and these risks build on each other, much like building blocks: the more blocks you try to stack, the more likely your tower will teeter and tumble. By actively eliminating potential fall risks, we are more likely to remain upright and steady, much like well-balanced meditative rock stacks.

Deprescribing can help us balance the benefit of useful medications with the risks of unexamined polypharmacy that can contribute to falls. Critically evaluating why a patient is taking specific medications can be an important step in finding this balance. Patients and health-care providers alike can resist this review, offering many barriers, excuses, and reasons why "that does not pertain to me" or "that does not pertain to that patient."

For example, Mr. Z, an older patient, was admitted to a hospital after a fall in the middle of the night. Mr. Z took both zolpidem (a prescription for insomnia) and a benzodiazepine (a prescription for anxiety/insomnia) at bedtime, so it's not surprising that he fell when he got up in the middle of the night. At the hospital, it was pointed out that both medications can increase the risk of falls, but the hospitalist said both were needed because Mr. Z could not fall asleep or stay asleep even with these medications. The question then is, why would Mr. Z continue these in the first place? They are not helping him sleep, so instead of being a therapeutic aid, the medications are simply increasing his fall risk.

Patients might say, "I need that," when a pharmacist or health-care provider recommends a change, even when their medications are potentially resulting in more harm than providing help. Why wait for the fall—or multiple falls—before taking action?

It is not uncommon for a patient to be on several medications that can increase the risk of falls. The Beers Criteria, STOPP, and CDC STEADI program, list many medications that can increase risk of falls. (More information on these lists is available in the Resources section.) Patients and health-care providers are encouraged to become familiar with these lists and consider the importance of fall prevention when prescribing or taking medications.

IN REAL LIFE

Falls and deprescribing

Mrs. D has a history of falls, including multiple times in one day. Her medication list follows: acetaminophen PM (for pain and sleep aid), atenolol (for heart rate and blood pressure), duloxetine (for depression and nerve pain), fentanyl (for pain), gabapentin (for neuropathy), glimepiride (for diabetes), lisinopril (for blood pressure), lovastatin (for cholesterol), mirtazapine (an antipsychotic / antidepressant), ropinirole (for restless leg), and trazodone (for insomnia and depression). Eight of these 11 medications can increase the risk of falls: acetaminophen PM, duloxetine, fentanyl, gabapentin, glimepiride, mirtazapine, ropinirole, and trazodone.

The remaining medications are not listed as high-fall-risk, but atenolol and lisinopril could contribute to a potential fall due to cardiovascular side effects, and lovastatin could contribute to a potential fall due to possible muscle weakness. In addition, many of these medications can cause cognitive deficits, which can cause a patient to become easily confused and take incorrect medications or incorrect dosages, possibly doubling up on medications by accident. You can see the culmination of possibilities that may cause harm for this patient and may be contributing to her many falls.

As has been pointed out throughout this book, the effects of medication can be additive, so a person's risk of falling increases when taking multiple medications that increase their risk of falls. Therefore, it's not necessarily one medication, but two or more medications together that could drive up fall risk. Using lowest possible doses and deprescribing unnecessary and duplicate medications can help lower the risk of falls.

Table 8.1 shows the precautions of Mrs. D's medication list based on various criteria. Perhaps deprescribing some medication by stopping and reducing others may be beneficial to reduce Mrs. D's falls. A health-care provider could first target acetaminophen PM, mirtazapine, or fentanyl, as these meds are each potentially inappropriate according to all three criteria reviewed.

Table 8.1

Mrs. D's Medications and Potential for Inappropriateness

Medication	Beers	STOPP	STEADI
Acetaminophen PM	x	x	x
Atenolol		x	x
Duloxetine	x		x
Fentanyl	x	x	x
Gabapentin	x		x
Glimepiride	x		
Lisinopril			x
Lovastatin			
Mirtazapine	x	x	x
Ropinirole			x
Trazodone			x

Newly prescribed medications can cause falls

Dicyclomine is a medication used for stomach irregularities such as nausea and irritable bowel. It's designed to keep your stomach moving in the right direction. Dicyclomine is not recommended for older adults and should be avoided, according to the Beer's Criteria. However, Mr. U, an older adult patient, was having irritable stomach issues and went to see his physician. The physician prescribed dicyclomine. The patient filled the prescription and began to take it according to the instructions.

Within three to five days of beginning the medication, Mr. U fell several times and became weak. The side effects of dicyclomine are significant—especially in older adults. It can be very drying, causing dry mouth, dry eyes, constipation, increased heart rate, weakness, confusion, and changes in balance. After it was noted that the Mr. U's falls might be due to the medication, the dicyclomine was stopped.

Reducing Readmissions

As seen above, medications may cause many admissions and readmissions to hospitals every year. Older adults with COPD and heart failure have a high rate of hospital readmission rates within 30 days of discharge. Readmission rates are also higher in the older population in general. Other risk factors for readmission of older adults include falls and polypharmacy. In a study that looked at hospital readmissions within 30 days of discharge, polypharmacy (extreme >10 meds) increased the risk of readmissions significantly.[59]

Readmissions can be avoided with a systematic review and advocacy for the patient. The *American Journal of Health Systems Pharmacy* has reported that a systematic approach reduced readmissions from 20% to 9.8%.[60]

1. **Reconcile the medication list.** Medications can be carried over on lists and never discontinued. When looking at electronic health records or pharmacy records, many prescriptions and

OTC medications remain on a patient's profile even when the product has been discontinued.

2. **Employ patient-centered education by the pharmacist during the hospital stay.** This education can be most helpful, as the patient or caregiver may be available and have the time to review the medications and report inconsistencies or other medications that may have been recently tried, started, or stopped by the patient.

3. **Ensure the patient has access to needed medications at discharge.** This can be a challenge especially if medications are expensive. Coverage, copayments, and insurance limitations, as well as transportation to pick up medications may all be barriers to a patient's receiving appropriate medications.

4. **Counsel the patient post-discharge.** Set up a check-in with the patient through programs such as visiting nurse and recommend that the patient speak with a pharmacist if more details are necessary.

5. **The patient remains home and avoids readmission.** The ultimate outcome when the steps are followed.

Action plans, as well as telehealth for specific needs, help to reduce potential readmissions. These plans were well in place prior to COVID, and now may become even more common, as the technology and comfort with telehealth appointments became commonplace during the epidemic.

Medications that need special attention

Some medications, especially insulin, levothyroxine, digoxin, and warfarin, have a higher risk of causing hospitalizations. These medications are more likely to cause problems because they have narrow therapeutic ranges, meaning a small change can have a big effect on the individual.

Diabetes medications. If you confuse medications and double up by accident, especially with a product that can cause low blood sugar, it may take extra time to increase the blood glucose level. If a person takes the normal dose of glyburide, then incorrectly thinks they have not taken the dose and takes another dose, hypoglycemia could occur. The same goes for insulin. If insulin is misdosed and more is injected, then a hypoglycemic effect may occur. Older adults who have poor eyesight (possibly due to diabetes) may incorrectly take a wrong dose. Sometimes insulins are confused; for example, the short-acting insulin is taken instead of the long-acting insulin, which is typically dosed higher as a 24-hour dose. This can pose a significant drop in blood glucose, which requires emergency intervention.

Levothyroxine. Small changes to this product, used for low thyroid, or hypothyroidism, can have a big impact for individuals. Side effects of too much thyroid medication include heart palpitations, anxiety, and insomnia, to name a few. Palpitations are a common reason people want to be seen by urgent care, emergency, or health-care providers. Thyroid stimulating hormone (TSH) is measured to determine treatment and to monitor treatment. The range is narrow, and hyperthyroid effects may be an issue when patients approach the lower side of the range. As older adults are more sensitive to cardiovascular side effects, being in the lower range of TSH values can be "too much" for an older adult. A higher level of TSH that is still in range may allow for fewer side effects and a safer level of treatment for the individual.

Digoxin. Used for heart failure and arrhythmias, levels of digoxin can easily become toxic, as determined by a blood test, causing vision changes, loss of appetite, stomach upset, dizziness, and confusion.

Warfarin. Used to reduce the risk of blood clots, warfarin effectiveness can vary due to medications, diet, and alcohol intake. Monitoring of warfarin is important to avoid under-target-dosing, which can cause blood clots, or over-target-dosing, which causes bleeding. The medication is adjusted according to blood clotting test checks, known as INR.

Choosing Wisely

Unfortunately, there are not always easy ways to rectify medication problems because there are not a lot of options to treat some patients, especially one with multiple illnesses. Sometimes doctors are choosing the "best" option when a "good" option is not available. This frequently occurs with treatments for chronic pain, Alzheimer's, depression, and anxiety.

But health-care providers should take care that they do not choose a "worse" option. And reaching for a new medication is not always the best choice either. Patients should seriously consider pursuing nonpharmacological options suggested by your health-care provider, such as music therapy, prayer, humor, meditation, yoga, strength training, pulmonary rehabilitation, cardiovascular rehabilitation, physical therapy, acupuncture, massage, behavioral therapy, and support groups.

In Part III we will continue to explore the process of deprescribing, focusing on the perspective of health-care providers and the obstacles that make deprescribing more difficult than it sounds.

Overview of Part II:

What Can We DO? Deprescribe to Optimize!

- Deprescribe to optimize (DO) is a thoughtful process that is shared between patients, caregivers, and health-care providers, including pharmacists, the medication experts.

- DO involves multiple conversations, action steps, monitoring, and documenting throughout the continuum of care.

- Prescribing and deprescribing use the same thought process: adding or subtracting a medication is an individualized, step-by-step process that requires monitoring to judge outcomes.

- The MedStrong Medication Optimization Plan (MOP) and the multiple MedStrong checklists provided in this book can help patients and providers successfully complete the deprescribing process. See appendix A for all the forms.

- Listing the medications you take and considering if each medication is effective, necessary, or added due to side effects is an important first step of MOP.

- Knowing the right questions to ask at the right time and in the right situation will help empower individuals to optimize their medications.

- Consider with your health-care providers if stopping, changing, or reducing a medication is a good therapeutic plan.

- Plan and be ready to monitor, document, and follow up on the steps in your plan.

- Know what's in your pill box. Being educated so that you can become your own best advocate is key to taking control of your health outcomes.

- As your body changes, consider the potential for side effects of various medications and the hazards of particular combinations.
- Deprescribing and optimizing medications can reduce hospitalizations, falls, and other adverse effects.

Many medications that are beneficial—even life-saving—for some people can be harmful to others. Prescribing and deprescribing should be part of a thoughtful, informed process with patients, caregivers, and health-care providers making decisions based on an individual's unique life circumstances. DO takes effort, but DO-ing keeps us enlightened, energized, accountable, and learning for the good of ourselves and others.

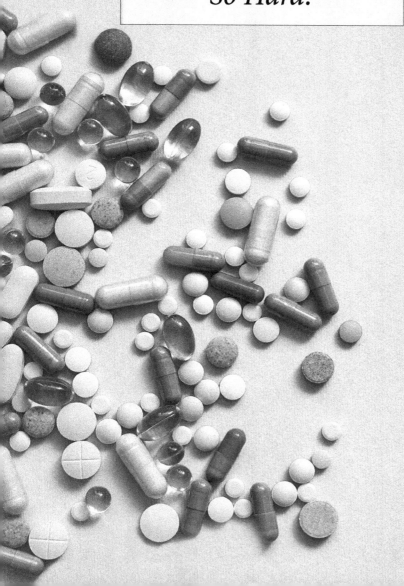

PART III

Why is Deprescribing So Hard?

CHAPTER 9

Deprescribing in a Prescribing World

Although the MedStrong Medication Optimization Plan (MOP) introduced in the previous chapters can help health-care providers navigate the deprescribing process, its primary purpose is to facilitate the journey for patients and caregivers. Fortunately, multiple models and strategies have been created for health-care providers, and several will be introduced in this chapter. There is not one particular deprescribing process considered the "gold standard" or "best option," so providers should adopt the variation that seems most natural or helpful for their practice. Though this chapter speaks more to health-care providers, consumers and caregivers can learn from this material, too. This chapter provides a perspective of deprescribing from the prescribers' point of view and barriers that affect both patients and providers.

As pointed out in chapter 4, "REMEDY: REthink the MEDs You take," the process of deprescribing should mimic the process of prescribing. Each patient case is reviewed through an individualized, step-by-step process that requires monitoring to evaluate whether a medication is necessary or can be deprescribed. When reviewing medications as a pharmacist, I use the Medication Appropriateness Index.[61,62] This list of 10 questions shown in table 9.1 serves as a map to make sense of medications being taken and helps me formulate questions to determine if the medication is indeed appropriate.

Table 9.1

Medication Appropriateness Index	
Indication	What is the medication being used for?
Effect	Is the medication effective for this use?
Dose	Is this dose correct?
Instructions	Are the directions correct?
Drug-drug Interactions	Are there drug-drug interactions of concern?
Drug-disease Interactions	Can the medication make another condition worse?
Duplications	Is the medication similar to another?
Practical	Can the patient use/take the medication properly?
Duration	How long should/how long has the drug been being taken?
Affordable	Is this the least expensive medication the patient could be taking for their condition?

If any of the questions elicit concerns about a medication, steps should be taken to further clarify the information. If it is determined a medication should be deprescribed, the next step is to develop a plan to help the patient and provider reach an agreeable protocol. Providers should consider what may need to be monitored and let the patient know what to expect during the process, including what changes they should consider "normal" and when to call the office with worrisome effects. A follow-up appointment may be necessary to determine if the deprescribing is appropriate.

How to Implement a Deprescribing Process

If someone has several medications, how does the health-care provider begin the deprescribing process? Which med (or meds) should be addressed first? Is there a method? Actually, health-care providers and researchers have proposed several methods and approaches in recent years. The first deprescribing process was outlined in 2003 as a four-step process.[63]

1. Review current meds.
2. Identify meds to stop, substitute, or reduce.
3. Plan a deprescribing regimen.
4. Frequently review and support patient.

A five-step approach was offered in a 2016 article in the *Journal of Pharmacy Practice and Research*.[64]

1. Identify if a patient is suitable for deprescribing. Not all patients have the buy-in to make a change, and not all will be willing to follow the deprescribing protocol. Many overprescribed medications can cause confusion or reduce cognition, making it difficult to have a patient realize the benefits of stopping a medication. In this situation, try to enlist caregivers to help support this endeavor.

2. Take a full medication history. It is best to be able to see the patient at home; however, this is not always possible. The full history will list all the patient's medications, including prescription, over-the-counter (OTC), supplements, and herbals. Ask the patient or caregiver how the product is actually taken and if it is currently being used.

3. Write up a medication withdrawal plan. Keep the individual in mind while creating this plan. How does the patient feel about it? What is most important for the patient? Determine which medications are appropriate, inappropriate, need further evaluation, or are not high priority. If you decide to discontinue medications, plan your next steps. Which one (or ones) first? Determining whether the patient is experiencing potential side effects may help you decide which drug to discontinue first. Can the medication be stopped abruptly or should it be tapered? What symptoms may return if the medication is still necessary? Also consider the general health and life expectancy of the patient when determining future benefit versus medication risks.

4. Stop one or more medications. Some medications should be stopped first to evaluate the effect on the patient so the next medication can be determined separately, and so on. For some medications— such as medications for pain, stomach upset, and anxiety—consider providing alternative or as-needed medications.

5. Monitor and follow up. Just as medications need to be monitored when they are prescribed, stopping medications also needs to be evaluated. For example, how often are on-demand medications being used during the process? Do adjustments to the process need to be slowed or adjustments made?

A similar process is recommended by the American College of Cardiology (ACC), which has noted that deprescribing may especially benefit older patients as treatment goals change.[65] The ACC Geriatric Council's five-step process emphasizes discussing priorities with the patient and family.

1. Review and reconcile medication.
2. Assess risk for adverse events from each medication.
3. Evaluate eligibility for discontinuation of each medication.
4. Discuss priorities for discontinuing drugs with the patient and their family.
5. Discontinue medications and monitor for events.

Yet another five-step process is recommended in a 2015 article, "Reducing Inappropriate Polypharmacy: The Process of Deprescribing."[66]

1. Ascertain all meds patient is taking and why.
2. Consider overall risk.

3. Assess each drug for eligibility to discontinue; consider indication, prescribing cascade, harm versus benefit, disease and symptom control, prevention benefit and patient longevity, and drug burden.
4. Prioritize drugs for discontinuation.
5. Implement a plan to discontinue and monitor.

This article, which includes a subheading with the words "Less Is More," emphasizes the number of unnecessary medicines seen in all areas of care, including the community, hospitals, and nursing homes. The unnecessary medications can include prescription and nonprescription medications, and the problem affects all ages.

The American Geriatric Society (AGS) has also provided guiding principles to aid in deprescribing.[67]

1. Obtain best possible medication history.
2. Identify inappropriate medications.
3. Determine medications to be withdrawn.
4. Plan and initiate withdrawal.
5. Monitor and document the process.

The AGS has also identified inappropriate medication categories that can be ideal targets for deprescribing, especially for older patients, as seen in table 9.2.

Table 9.2

Potentially Inappropriate Meds for Older Adults

Potential Innapropriate Category	Example
Original indication (health concern) no longer applies	During a hospitalization, the patient was given a medication, such as a proton pump inhibitor (e.g., omeprazole), to prevent gastric acid and ulcers while hospitalized. The patient is still taking the medication a year later, without an indication or need for the med.

Potential Innapropriate Category	Example
Drug-drug interactions	A patient is taking amlodipine for blood pressure and simvastatin 40mg for cholesterol. Since amlodipine can increase the drug availability of simvastatin, it is recommended that the simvastatin be reduced to 20mg to reduce the drug-drug interaction and potential muscle ache and pain side effects the patient may encounter or already experience.
Drug-disease interactions	A patient experiences knee pain from walking and decides to take ibuprofen. The patient has heart failure and begins to retain fluids, experiences swollen ankles, and becomes short of breath. The ibuprofen has caused an exacerbation of heart failure. Providers should advise patients to avoid ibuprofen and similar products for future episodes of pain and make recommendations about what can be taken.
Inappropriate treatment for patient life expectancy	An 85-year-old patient with type 2 diabetes is experiencing many episodes of low blood sugar (hypoglycemia). His HgA1c is 7%. The provider decides to stop one of the medications used to treat diabetes and tells patient A1c could go as high as 8.5% without concern. Although lower A1c levels are important in younger patients to protect smaller blood vessels, the higher A1c is less risky than hypoglycemic (low blood sugar) episodes in older patients.

Potential Innapropriate Category	Example
Medication no longer aligns with goals	A patient would prefer to be on less medication, experience fewer side effects, and have a better daily quality of life than be on higher doses at thera-peutic goals, which could extend life but leave them unable to enjoy their favorite activities.
Medication poses high risk of falls / traffic accidents	Zolpidem, used for sleep, can cause falls, traffic accidents, and confusion, especially in older patients. Advise patient to reduce caffeine and chocolate, exercise regularly, and avoid electronics at bedtime to improve sleep and eliminate need for zolpidem at bedtime.
Experencing an adverse effect	A patient being treated for pain with tramadol has a seizure. Tramadol should be stopped, as it can lower seizure threshold. Better to deprescribe a medication than to add medications for a side effect.

The Targeted Approach

Another approach to deprescribing is to begin by targeting one group of health issues. For example, begin with medications that have significant side effects, such as anticholinergics, increased risk of falls, or cognition effects. Next, target legacy prescriptions: medications that should be prescribed only for a moderate length of time, not indefinitely. Or review specific medications first, such as antiseizure meds, proton pump inhibitors (PPIs), or gabapentin. This approach can be especially beneficial when a provider is hindered by time constraints. The categories illustrated in table 9.2 can be good areas to target in this approach.

A Closer Look: Insomnia Medications

An article highlighting an interview with Dr. Kevin Pottie, associate professor of the Departments of Family Medicine and Epidemiology & Community Medicine at the University of Ottawa, offers glimpses of the problems of polypharmacy for insomnia treatment.[68] Insomnia medications can cause cognitive impairment, falls, and traffic accidents. Not only that, their effectiveness over a long period of time is questionable.

There are also confusing dosing restrictions of some medications for insomnia, such as zolpidem. Zolpidem should be dosed at 5 mg at bedtime for women and all older adults regardless of gender, and dosed at 10 mg at bedtime for younger adult males. The use of these medications in older adults is cautioned against in many of the criteria available including the Beers Criteria, STOPP and START, CDC-STEADI, and Choosing Wisely.

If someone really cannot sleep, what should be done for them? More and more studies are showing the benefits of nonmedication approaches, such as encouraging better sleep hygiene and counseling, including cognitive behavior therapy. Improving sleep hygiene may include reducing foods and activities that may cause insomnia, such as caffeine and chocolate, and avoiding napping during the day and screen time later in the day or evening.

Dr. Pottie mentions that instead of getting caught in the cycle of finding a medication to treat a patient's insomnia, health-care providers should first review current medications that may be causing the insomnia.

It could be the timing of medications or some other underlying issue such as pain, sleep apnea, or anxiety that could be keeping the patient awake.

Pause and Monitor

Pause and monitor is another approach to deprescribing, and it calls for patients and prescribers to work together to decide if a medication is actually necessary, especially if there is question of risk versus benefit. Pause and monitor allows both parties to commit to the idea of deprescribing, while also committing to follow up to determine the results.[69] This process can be especially helpful when either the patient or the provider is leery about stopping a medication. Including a "pause and monitor" clause in any deprescribing approach may make it easier for the patient and provider to share in the decision-making process.

Another way providers can help make the deprescribing process easier is by asking patients questions that ensure they are involved in the process. These questions include

- What matters to you?
- Is deprescribing something you would consider?
- What medications are important to you and why?
- What options would you like to have?

Team Approach

All of these approaches demonstrate that deprescribing should be an individualized, multilayer process that involves cooperation between the patient, providers, and caregivers. This cooperation plays a key role in whether the deprescribing process succeeds.

Think about it: if a patient, caregiver, or pharmacist approaches a doctor about deprescribing and the doctor dismisses the request without a good explanation, then they are not working as a team. If a doctor makes an effort to inform the pharmacy that a medication was deprescribed, but the pharmacy does not update the patient's records and continues to make medication refills available, then the team approach has been dismissed. Because there are so many scenarios that can stop deprescribing in its tracks, it sometimes requires multiple attempts to succeed.

The deprescribing process should be a pragmatic, methodical, and monitored team effort, and if one member or part of the team effort breaks down, the whole process can also break down. Primary care providers, specialists, and pharmacists all need to be on board, willing to communicate, and able to make changes effectively. Without a team effort, one provider may recommend a change that does not get carried forth.

For example, automatic prescription refills can derail a deprescribing effort. A provider tells a patient to stop taking a medication, but a refill of the medication becomes available at the pharmacy a few weeks later. The patient may become confused and think the doctor ordered the medication again. Health-care providers need to be able to communicate changes to multiple team members to ensure the changes are made in all arms of the system, rather than expecting the patient to make the system work.

Changing the Culture

The growing evidence for the benefits of deprescribing in health outcomes, quality of life, and cost containment calls for a cultural change that will expect deprescribing to be integrated into the process the moment a medication is prescribed. "Life-long medications" should be a thing of the past.[70] Instead, providers should establish a time span to review medications and either continue therapy or stop therapy as part of the health-care protocol. Adding a commitment to deprescribing should be considered in every patient encounter.

Deprescribing does not mean health-care providers give up on their patients, stop all their medications, and stop prescribing for preventive purposes. Instead, deprescribing is another way of managing risks and benefits while considering many factors that influence good medicine. It takes skill to look at a patient's health changes and realize the moment when a medicine is no longer efficacious or when it begins to pose an unacceptable risk or burden.

Currently, there is minimal professional guidance to help health-care providers know when to stop medications or how to determine whether harm may occur over time if medications are or are not stopped. Studies are necessary to evaluate these outcomes, but who should be responsible for studying these factors? Will a manufacturer be on board with studying the best ways to stop medications? Should we have both prescribing information and deprescribing information for all medications?

What about the patient goals within these guidelines? When is it time to stop a medication for a patient? Do we wait for the hospitalization, the fall, the adverse event before we intervene? Perhaps there needs to be a deprescribing treatment plan within the treatment guidelines, but further study is needed before that can be done.

Health-care providers do not want to remove medications that are providing benefit and certainly do not want to swing the pendulum from overtreatment to undertreatment. Taking small steps, reevaluating, and monitoring the patient throughout the deprescribing process does take time, but it allows for intervention if necessary.

Providers should also recognize that in the process of deprescribing, "no change" in how the patient is doing can be a good outcome, which is an odd idea for medical professionals accustomed to trying to effect a change. But a patient who stops taking a medication and experiences no change in a condition may very well be counted as a successful deprescribing outcome.

Many medications are intended for chronic, indefinite use; however, labeling a medication as a "lifetime" medication can be inappropriate. As suggested in the "Reducing Inappropriate Polypharmacy" article, medications should be labeled "best before" and then reevaluated for continuation after that date.[71] When counseling patients, health-care providers can tell them that certain medications may need to be taken indefinitely but also warn them that there may very well be a time when discontinuation is warranted.

Providers and patients alike can use the MedStrong Annual Physical Med Checklist (see figure 9.3 and also appendix A) to make this process easier. Each line includes a check box to "Deprescribe" or "Continue," to help foster the idea of thoughtfully reviewing all medications and considering whether it's time to deprescribe.

Figure 9.3

MedStrong Annual Physical Med Checklist

My Medication and Strength	How Taken & When	Reason for the Medication	ACTION - Check the Box That Applies	
			Deprescribe	Continue

Changes to medication reviews in hospitals could benefit patients. At most emergency departments and hospitals, medication reviews are generally referred to as a "med-rec" or medication reconciliation. The end product is usually an updated list of medications a patient may have been taking prior to the hospital visit. Ideally, this list would be used to provide a true medication review, although that would require a cultural shift at most hospitals. Changing "med-rec" to "med-rev" and promoting a routine deprescribing process will require more time and attention, but such a change could result in better patient outcomes and reduced readmissions.

How can health-care providers work toward a true "med-rev" system? The processes and approaches described in this chapter offer good starting points. Another way to jumpstart the deprescribing process is to honestly examine the difficulties and address the barriers for both patients and health-care providers.

As we have seen, the benefits of deprescribing can include a lower pill burden; fewer side effects and drug interactions; optimization of medications; potential reduction of fall risks, geriatric syndromes, inappropriate medications, hospitalizations due to medication adverse events, and health-care costs; and improved patient satisfaction, adherence to medications, and quality of life.[72]

With so many benefits, it seems like deprescribing would be an easy sell to everyone involved. Unfortunately, the barriers are just as abundant. Let's review those barriers and examine how the barriers could be addressed and changed.

Barriers to Deprescribing

One of the most important—and perhaps one of the most complicated—factors in deprescribing is determining exactly what medications a patient is taking. Researchers in one study, "Stopping Inappropriate Medicines in the Outpatient Setting,"noted that gathering an updated medication record can be challenging.[73]

In this study, a pilot to review STOPIT (Screening Tool for Older People's Inappropriate Treatment), patients' medication histories were gathered from several sources, especially in outpatient settings.

Medication history sources are derived from patient or caregiver memory, a printout from a primary care office or pharmacy/pharmacies, charts from nursing homes, or discharge summaries from a hospitalization. Some patients bring handwritten lists of their medications, while others bring the medications themselves. Other patients cannot remember the names of medications they take nor when or how often they are supposed to take them.

Evaluating a patient's medications is only part of the burden; health-care providers also need to evaluate a patient's current health status to make sure medications are not being prescribed to treat a condition that no longer needs to be treated. In "Undiagnosing to Prevent Overprescribing," the authors note that some disease states may remain on a patient's health record as active issues even if the problem has been addressed or resolved through other steps, such as lifestyle changes, smoking cessation, or stress reduction.[74]

Medications to treat those now-resolved health conditions may continue to be prescribed because practitioners are trying to ensure that all medical conditions are being treated appropriately and according to guidelines. So, a failure to fully update a patient's health records when a condition is no longer clinically relevant or in need of medical treatment can lead to overprescribing.

A lack of guidelines for deprescribing can also make some health-care providers reluctant to tackle the process. Although it is easy to find treatment guidelines and medication continuation information, guidelines for reducing or stopping medication are limited.

However, a process called ERASE can be used as a systematic means to reducing polypharmacy and overprescribing. ERASE stands for "Evaluate diagnoses through the consideration of Resolved conditions, Ageing normally and Selecting appropriate targets to

Eliminate unnecessary diagnoses and associated medicines."[75] This unique concept can assist health-care providers in reducing multiple diagnoses that complicate the deprescribing process, including medical-cultural factors and new diagnosis levels, for example "pre-diabetes."

Moving on through the barriers, we will explore prescriber barriers and patient barriers and learn how educating ourselves— whether we are the patient, caregiver, or prescriber—is paramount to navigating the process successfully.

Prescriber Barriers

Uncertainty

The study "Self-Efficacy for Deprescribing: A Survey for Health Care Professionals Using Evidence-Based Deprescribing Guidelines," notes that self-efficacy may be a barrier to deprescribing for some prescribers.[76] Self-efficacy refers to the personal judgment of one's ability to fulfill a function based on knowledge, attitude, cognitive skills, and the circumstance. Health-care providers who practice in long-term care have more experience in the area of deprescribing, and, in surveys, they expressed more self-efficacy in deprescribing than did family health team prescribers, who may not be as inclined to deprescribe on a regular basis.

However, prescribers become more comfortable with deprescribing when guidelines to the process are provided as a tool. Guidelines are the result of evidence-based medicine, practice-based goals of health care, and truly the cornerstone of treatment and treatment decisions. However, without guidelines, practitioners may fear they do not have evidence to support their decision if nontreatment becomes an issue and litigation is pursued. In our culture of litigation, this can certainly impose a barrier.

Many prescribers may know that deprescribing is appropriate but may be uncertain how to implement it and of the process. Creating and promoting better guidelines for deprescribing would help health-care providers become more comfortable with the process. Some medical questionnaires that may be incorporated to help providers better understand the benefit or harm of deprescribing include the cognitive function test Mini Mental Status Examination (MMSE), physical function Modified Barthel Index (MBI), bowel function assessment (RACF), self-reported Quality of Life in Alzheimer's Disease (QOLAD), self-reported health (EQ-5D), and self-assessment Pittsburg Sleep Quality Index (PSQI).

A Closer Look: Educating Health-Care Providers

Health-care professionals are rarely taught how to reduce medications. Evidence for reducing medications is in its infancy. Treatment guidelines rarely discuss reducing medications. This perfect storm of unavailable information, lack of training, and absence of evidence prohibit the standard practice of deprescribing.

More education, better guidelines, increased research and advocacy, and new policies to recognize the value of pharmacists and health-care providers in this important aspect of care can help deprescribing become more mainstream. Advocates believe health-care professionals should learn about deprescribing throughout their curriculum in order to have a continual practice of prescribing and deprescribing along the entire continuum of care. A commitment to this process has already begun in some places.

Australia, Canada, and the United States have networks to promote the awareness, research, and advocacy of deprescribing. The International Group for Reducing Inappropriate Medication Use and Polypharmacy addresses deprescribing as a global concern. Choosing Wisely is another international awareness organization that reviews medications, medical tests, treatments, and procedures that may be deemed unnecessary.

Manufacturers study dose outcomes, including efficacy and safety of medications, and provide maximum dosing advice and distribute other warnings and concerns about appropriate dosing for kidney and liver function. However, there is currently no requirement to provide advice for reducing or stopping medications, although some medications do offer such guidance. Providing education and information within drug monographs would be helpful, although further study of a medication may be needed to determine these parameters.

∽

Benefit-versus-harm questions

Poor outcomes or potential harms may occur with deprescribing, especially if a medication that needs to be tapered is stopped too suddenly, which may result in withdrawal reactions, changes in other medications (pharmacokinetic and pharmacodynamics), or a return of symptoms of the health condition.[77] Medications that may cause withdrawal reactions include beta-blockers, antidepressants, antianxiety, opioids, and proton pump inhibitors (PPIs), to name a few.

Drug-drug interactions that cause medications to compete for metabolism or receptors may cause increased or decreased amounts of the medication in the body. Medications that increase or decrease electrolytes may affect the electrolyte balance, causing confusion, falls, and weakness. Lastly, a return of the health condition may be detrimental, as in seizure or depression relapses, for example.

However, one may not be able to measure the harm or benefit of stopping a preventative medication unless it is stopped. For all these reasons, health-care providers should work with patients to monitor changes and to taper or change medications in a methodical, safe, manner.

Difficult process

"Knowledge and Willingness of Physicians about Deprescribing Among Older Patients: A Qualitative Study," conducted in Saudi Arabia, highlights barriers to deprescribing that appear to be no different in other parts of the world.[78] The study notes that deprescribing is time-consuming and exacerbated by a lack of communication between physicians and specialists. Some physicians may not know the provider of a certain prescription and will not take the time to find out, nor be the one to deprescribe the medication.

In the article "Undoing What We've Done: Why Deprescribing Is So Difficult," Dr. P. A. Masters reviews a medication list of one patient with a few health conditions.[79] The patient states she cannot keep the 15 medications straight, does not feel well on all the medicines, and spends too much money. Dr. Masters notices right away that some medications are also on the AGS Beers Criteria and may be potentially inappropriate for this patient.

The doctor then poses the tough questions as to why patients end up on so many meds that can cause harm; provide little to no benefit for a particular patient; and can lead to adverse reactions, falls, hospital admissions, and even death? Why are too many medications prescribed in the first place, and why is it not standard for prescribers to stop or reduce medicines?

Some answers may lie in the disease-state guidelines. If patients are being treated per disease and each disease guideline, multiple medications may easily be added to a patient's med list, especially since many patients are followed by more than one doctor who may end up adding medications to treat the side effects of medicines prescribed by other doctors. It can be easier to continue drug therapy, as patients may offer less resistance.

Dr. Masters proposes that the solution can be a team effort, where all prescribers in all areas of care—including primary, specialists, hospitalist, emergency—take the opportunity to think about the prescribing practices for a patient. Prescribers can pose these questions regarding need of medications:

- Is there truly an indication for the medication?
- If so, how will it fit into the overall context of the patient's treatment to minimize drug interactions and adverse side effects?
- What is the duration of therapy?
- If the drug regimen is changed, will it really benefit the patient, and can the patient afford the medicine?
- If there is a change, is it temporary or indefinite?
- How can we communicate this so that we all know the rationale of these changes, the plans, and details of the treatment?

Back to Dr. Master's patient: the physician believed that up to 12 of her medications were most likely added to address side effects of other medications and that the patient could reasonably reduce her medications down to three. The patient was excited about this and ready to begin what could be a long process to make all the changes.

Patient Barriers

Patient barriers to deprescribing are very real. Many fear the return or worsening of a medical condition. Some have had a poor experience when trying to stop medications previously. Some caregivers may object to the planned change for their loved ones or clients or may want the health-care provider to come up with a new or better medication to try for a particular condition. Other barriers include patients who face multiple illnesses and morbidities; many of them are being treated by multiple providers and may be reluctant to trust any one doctor or specialist to address all their medications.[80] Education and communication are key in addressing the concerns of patients and caregivers through this process.

When I approached older adults at an outreach program or at the pharmacy, where I was dispensing prescriptions for over 20 years, too many times I ran into a wall the patient erected to prevent a medication review. I have heard countless times, "My doctor checks all my medications." I'm not saying that's not true, but is the doctor considering all the medications, by all the specialists, plus all the OTC products, supplements, and herbals you may be taking? Is your doctor reviewing for potential side effects, and are you reporting all your side effects, such as falls, dizzy spells, and dry mouth? Remember medication reviews take time and are not a one-time-only conversation. Why not ask the medication expert, your pharmacist, for their educated opinion? These conversations can help facilitate effective conversations with your health-care providers, as I have heard many times from those that did take the time to review their medications with me.

Prescribers and patients should be ready to discuss the fears and concerns of patients or caregivers when approaching the deprescribing process. Be willing to share and consider data and to talk about life expectancy and the patient experience of deprescribing, such as potential withdrawal syndromes or condition relapses—but also the potential of improved health and well-being.

Shared decision-making may also alleviate some of these barriers. Take a team approach with all of a patient's specialists, pharmacists, and caregivers to provide best guidance and action and to address a patient's fears and preferences. Such an approach may help ease patients' resistance to deprescribing.

Providers may also choose to target risk-reducing medications, such as aspirin, statins, bisphosphonates, antihypertensives, and vitamins, to deprescribe first. Patients do not necessarily "feel" the benefit of these medications so may be less reluctant to forego them.

Geriatricians Tackle the Barriers

Geriatricians are frequently more practiced in tackling the deprescribing process than are other health-care providers. Geriatricians are very practical about patient medications, experiences, adherence to medications, needs of the patient, and ease of administration for the caregivers. They assess patients and critically evaluate their medications for benefit versus harm and provide a simplified approach for all involved in the care of the individual.

I spoke with Dr. Anthony Zizza, a geriatrician and senior medical officer of Landmark Health, regarding deprescribing techniques, and he explained that quick wins help health-care providers gain patients' trust and cooperation. It is better to make some smaller changes at first, especially those that may not need to be tapered, he said, noting that his patients rarely need to go back on the full strength of medication.

After deprescribing, Dr. Zizza said, his patients overwhelmingly feel better. They are moving better, sleeping better, enjoying a better quality of life, and thinking better! Too many doctors hear the woes of patients, especially older patients, and add on more medications. But many doctors who deprescribe hear and see how much better patients feel without a medication.

Some geriatrician offices are changing the way they practice and seeing patients in their homes, reducing barriers that make it hard for patients to get to an appointment. In this type of health-care group, the doctors, nurses, social workers, and case managers are always available and make house calls. In the world of deprescribing, this is an excellent way to see exactly what is happening in the home, such as how medications are managed, the OTC meds that are readily available to the patient, and safety measures / concerns. The home visits are more accessible than seeing a doctor at the office, allowing for increased check-in and follow-up and potentially a continuous attempt of deprescribing. Because patients are typically seen sooner, they may avoid needing urgent or emergent care.

Education Can Break Down Barriers

A study recording some of the thoughts, ideas, and actions of patients, caregivers, and providers about a prescribing cascade in an Alzheimer's patient[81] revealed how some practices can combat that process and encourage deprescribing. The providers freely admitted that they were likely to ignore a generalized letter from an insurance company but more likely to consider a specific communication about a particular patient and that patient's medication. And they would be even more likely to respond and act on a prescribing cascade if the patient or caregiver raised specific information or questions.

This study truly emphasizes the importance of bringing education about deprescribing (yes, that's right, including this very book in your hands!) directly to health-care consumers and caregivers—like you! Asking direct, informed questions definitely increases the likelihood that your provider will address your concerns and be willing to discuss deprescribing.

The deprescribing process and communication can also differ depending on ethnicity and race, as can be seen in the 2020 study "Designing a Primary Care-Based Deprescribing Intervention for Patients with Dementia and Multiple Chronic Conditions."[82] Prescribers, patients, and caregivers discussed how deprescribing is perceived and what is most helpful; and cultural perceptions, trust, and communication played important roles in the findings. Trust is important for all patients, independent of ethnicity and race. As long as there is trust with the physician, patients are more likely to engage in deprescribing. However, participants who identified as Hispanic in the study noted that language barriers and time constraints reduce their likelihood of accepting deprescribing.

One of the best ways to overcome the reluctance of patients or caregivers to participate in deprescribing is to educate them about the benefits and the harms of all their medications and to make the patients feel they are part of a team. Patients also feel better when there is follow-through, including telehealth visits and follow-up phone calls.

Deprescribing is so specific to individuals and includes so many variables that it can be difficult to gather evidence about its effectiveness.[83] A medicine that one patient needs to survive may in turn be causing side effects or drug interactions that limit the quality of life for another person. Stopping a medication for a cohort of patients to determine whether there is a benefit or harm is not an ideal study approach. This limitation presents a barrier for prescribers and patients.

To help overcome that barrier, prescribing and deprescribing can be viewed as individualized evidence-gathering missions. When starting a new medication, providers and patients can view that new drug as more of a trial to determine its benefits rather than a permanent addition to the patient's pillbox. The same attitude can be used when deprescribing: providers and patients might be more willing to enter the deprescribing process if they consider it more of a trial than a permanent elimination.

Statistics show that more than half of hospital admissions for adverse drug reactions occur for people 65 years of age and older.[84] Increasing public awareness about deprescribing can be a vital step in reducing that number by changing the culture of our overmedicated world, especially for older adults.

And research shows that doctors and other health-care providers play a vital role in that education process. Although less than 20% of older people agree they may be taking medications they no longer need, more than 90% would be willing to reduce medications if they were told by a physician that it was safe to do so.

I can certainly verify that a physician's opinion about reducing or stopping a medication carries tremendous weight for most patients.

For years, I have seen my parents ebb and flow with various medication-related side effects. I have sometimes suggested that they may need to stop taking a medication or suggested they should let the doctor know about a particular issue. But my suggestions are never as revered as the physician's, regardless of my professional qualifications and experience in this area. So when their doctor suggests they reduce a medication, I always act surprised, smile, and state, "That's a great idea!" And I am pleased that at least I have planted a seed.

A pharmacist can be the best option to provide information to both patients and prescribers. They are your central point between patients and prescribers, at least for medication purposes, and can provide medication therapy management. Many pharmacists are the most accessible health-care team member, even as they play many roles and provide many functions.

Pharmacists can assist with questions about prescription and nonprescription medications, counsel patients on potential side effects and drug interactions, describe how the medication is supposed to help, and give advice about how to take or use a medication. Pharmacists can help patients with their medication lists and scheduling of medications, and suggest questions that patients should ask their providers. Pharmacists also can assist with insurance and coverage issues and offer alternative medications that may be safer and more affordable yet still provide the intended outcome. Pharmacists also provide information to prescribers on drug interactions, drug duplications, dosing parameters, and clinical questions. Pharmacists are truly key members of the health-care team and key players in raising awareness about deprescribing and educating patients and prescribers about its benefits.

It's obvious that health-care providers have tremendous power to promote deprescribing as a healthy change in our overmedicated culture. But institutions and industry have a role to play, too, as we will see in the next chapter.

CHAPTER 10

Pharma Fails

THROUGHOUT MUCH OF THIS BOOK, we have reviewed the roles that patients, caregivers, pharmacists, and providers play in polypharmacy and the deprescribing process; but individuals are only part of the health-care picture. The pharmaceutical industry, including pharmacy chains and pharmaceutical manufacturers; and the insurance sector, including private, state, and government-run insurances, play large roles in the way medication is prescribed and dispensed in the United States. Just like the patients, caregivers, and prescribers, they also bear some of the polypharmacy burden and should share in the responsibility of making deprescribing easier and safer. In this chapter, we will examine some of the barriers that can make polypharmacy and the deprescribing process more difficult than it should be.

Brand-Name Extensions

Have you heard about brand-name extensions? As if over-the-counter (OTC) medications were not confusing enough, your drugstore shelves are now crowded with brand-name products followed by letters, such as DM, CF, PM, AM, to specify what is inside. They can be very confusing and even overlooked when selecting a product. Have you ever gone to the store to get some Advil or Tylenol for your headache and realized when you got home that you had grabbed the Advil PM or Tylenol PM by mistake?

Even trickier: some brand-name extension products do not even contain the original medication at all. Zantac originally hit shelves with the active ingredient ranitidine, but that product was taken off the market. However, today you can find Zantac 360° on the shelves, although its active ingredient is famotidine. Confused? You should be!

Claritin has done similar things with allergy medicine. Loratadine is the active ingredient in the oral allergy medication sold under the brand name Claritin. But ketotifen is the active ingredient in Claritin eyedrops, which are labeled as "allergy eye itch relief." It is truly amazing that this kind of branding is allowed, because it makes it so hard for consumers to know how to recognize when products change or to realize that ingredients in these OTC products can interact with their other medications. In pharmacy school, we are constantly reminded to beware of look-a-like, sound-a-like medications that could be easily mixed up and accidently dispensed incorrectly. How can untrained consumers be expected to keep up with all the look-a-like, sound-a-like OTC products?

Now let's take this a step further. When you list your OTC products on your MedStrong Medication list, what if you write Zantac but leave off the 360°? What about Claritin? Do you specify whether you are taking Claritin or Claritin D? Or Claritin eyedrops? All have different ingredients that can make a difference in what your health-care providers know about the possibility of drug interactions or side effects.

IN REAL LIFE

Brand-name extensions can cause problems, especially for older patients, as you can see from these examples.

Mrs. G had been admitted to the hospital twice in a short time period after falling. When she was admitted to the hospital, her kidney function was poor at admission, both times, but it had returned to normal by the time of discharge. The pharmacists found this odd enough to ask about what medications she was taking at home. She mentioned that she took Excedrin if she experienced a migraine that was resistant to her prescription migraine products. The pharmacist, knowing there are many OTC Excedrin products, pressed the patient for more details. Mrs. G then specified that she would take Excedrin Extra Strength, every 6 hours for a number of days in a row. This one detail helped explain the problem: the combination of medications was affecting her kidney function, causing medications to build up in her system and leading to falls. Had Mrs. G not been pressed for more specifics, the underlying medication culprit might have been overlooked.

Mr. N was also falling and getting easily confused. During a home visit, the pharmacist discovered that he had been taking Tylenol PM instead of regular Tylenol. Tylenol PM contains diphenhydramine, an antihistamine that causes sleepiness and is used as a sleep aid.[85] Mr. N was taking Tylenol PM several times a day, which was leading to his falls and confusion.

These two examples show how easily brand-name extensions can lead to problems. But these kinds of mix-ups are truly health system issues. If we have evidence that such a mix-up has happened once, there are probably many other cases that have not been detected or recorded.

Companies choose brand-name extensions because brand-name recognition makes it easier to market new products. But do they also recognize the dangers they are posing to patients who end up falling or hospitalized, or possibly experiencing a drug-drug interaction or drug-disease interaction because a product's brand name obscures its active ingredients?

Auto-Refills: A Help or a Hazard?

There are (at least) two sides to every story. A saying that always makes me laugh is "There are two sides to every story, then there is the real story!" Auto-refill is a good example of this adage. Having prescriptions set to auto-refill can be convenient and very helpful for individuals who have a hard time remembering to order refills before they run out of meds they desperately need. On the other hand, auto-refills can sometimes be filled when a medication should no longer be taken.

Of course, prescriptions do expire over time, depending in part on the medication, and in the United States, in which state the pharmacy is located.[86] Some states allow a prescription to be on auto-refill for up to two years; others may allow 15–18 months; and others, 12 months. Controlled medications (medications that can be addicting or abused) can have refills, depending upon the class, for up to six months, while others may be filled only once.

But what happens when a health-care provider decides to remove a long-term prescription from a patient's regimen? The doctor may tell the patient not to refill the medication, but will the patient remember to remove that prescription from auto-refill, especially if it is on a two-year cycle or if it has been filled or transferred to another pharmacy? Auto-refill makes it far too easy for a prescription to be continued and then renewed, even though the prescriber thought it had been discontinued long ago.

And how easily can pharmacists recognize that a medication has been discontinued if the patient—or auto-fill system—sends a refill request? I have seen prescribers write, "Do not fill unless the patient calls," "Place on hold until needed," or, for a new prescription strength, to "Cancel all previous prescriptions." But if that prescription note is forwarded to only one pharmacy, what happens to refills that may still be available at other pharmacies?

Medication Review Shortfalls

Medication reviews are an important aspect of your health care. These reviews may be conducted at your yearly physical, and some insurers may allow medication reviews to be conducted at your pharmacy or over the telephone with a health-care provider of the insurance company. Such reviews can be useful, but limited allocation of time and uneven insurance coverage can undermine the review process.

How much time is being allocated for the medicine review? Is your pharmacist or health-care provider or insurance representative taking the time to hear about all your OTC medications and all the prescriptions written by another doctor or filled at a different pharmacy? Does your provider know that your insurance insists you take a similar generic medication rather than the drug that was ordered? Patients may find their insurance will allow for a medication review one year, but they may no longer meet the qualifications a subsequent year.

Instead of relying on formal medication reviews, it might be better if patients and health-care providers review medications and make needed adjustments at every visit or encounter. Providers and patients should discuss this question: "Have I had to take any over-the-counter medications since my last visit?" This question can help you and your provider uncover issues you have had to treat, such as headaches, constipation, diarrhea, heartburn, runny nose, dry eyes, or pain. All of these conditions could be caused by a medication you are taking, even one that you have been taking for some time. Discussing these issues can help lead to a more thorough medication review.

Medication Therapy Management: Benefits and Limitations

Medication therapy management (MTM) is a process that pharmacists and health-care providers can follow to optimize individual medication lists by providing comprehensive reviews.

There are five key elements of MTM as structured by the American Pharmacists Association and National Association of Chain Drug Stores Foundation:[87]

1. Medication therapy review
2. Personal medication record
3. Medication-related action plan
4. Intervention and referrals
5. Documentation and follow-up

For billing purposes, MTM providers must use particular forms for their patients who qualify for these services. Although the MedStrong Medication Optimization Plan (MOP) introduced in this book cannot be submitted as MTM documentation, it can help patients and providers address all of the MTM elements, especially if patients and providers use the various forms to keep track of medications and changes in medications.

In a medication review, pharmacists and health-care providers get a better understanding of a patient's goals, overall health status, and any health literacy issues or financial issues that may make it hard for a patient to afford or correctly use a particular medication. It also gives providers a chance to determine whether a medication may be related to a patient's health concerns—even when the patient may have no idea that a medication may be causing problems.

The medication-related action plan sets up the patient to take action steps agreed upon by the patient and provider, so shared decision-making occurs in this step. Some action steps may be to take a medication at a different time for better outcomes or fewer adverse effects. Other action steps may address lifestyle changes, dietary modifications, improving sleep quality, and managing anxiety, to name a few.

If necessary, referrals are suggested to other health-care providers such as nutritionists or physical or occupational therapists. Or an individual may be encouraged to join an older adult center that has programs such as Matter of Balance, tai chi, walking groups, or exercise groups for reducing falls, building strength, and improving balance.

Documentation and follow-up are vital to the success of MTM, and shortcomings in either of those areas can undermine its effectiveness. Without the correct record-keeping or follow-through, it may be difficult for the MTM provider to bill for services or communicate with other health-care providers.

Problems can occur when medication records are incomplete or not updated. For example, many patients hand me a medication list to review and then proceed to tell me that a certain medication has been changed or stopped or that there is a new one that "I cannot remember the name of, and I have not added it to the list."

Other limitations to MTM rise from the complexities imposed by insurers. Medicare Part D insurance companies need to provide MTM per the guidelines of the Centers for Medicare and Medicaid Services. However, insurance companies are allowed to set their own eligibility guidelines. So, the insurance company determines the number of chronic conditions needed for MTM, and many require three from a predetermined list of conditions per the insurance company. If you have three conditions, but one of your conditions is not on the list, then you would not qualify for the service.

Other criteria include a particular number of medications, and that number can also vary. Many insurance companies require a person to be taking eight medications to be eligible for an MTM management review. Another criterion the company sets is the cost of the medications. So, if you do have three conditions that match the insurer's list of conditions and you do take eight medications but you take lower-cost generics, you still may not be eligible for MTM services. Furthermore, you may meet the criteria one year but not the next, especially if your medications are changed to lower-cost generics.

Of course, lower-cost medications can still cause side effects; be duplicated; have adverse interactions; cause falls, confusion, incontinence, and weakness, so limiting MTM reviews based on the price of medications makes little sense. Because we cannot count on the health system to provide the medication reviews we may need, we must rely on advocating for ourselves and those we care for as they age.

IN REAL LIFE

Timing is everything.

I sat down with Mrs. T at a community program to provide a medication review and initiate an MTM process. She had provided all of her medications in a brown bag, and I began to review her medications one by one. We discussed why she was taking each medication and how she was taking it. We spoke about how she felt throughout the day, and I asked if she had any issues or concerns. Mrs. T told me she often did not feel well later in the afternoon and was experiencing falls.

I looked back over her medications and asked when she was taking her two daily doses of glyburide. She explained that she took her first dose in the morning with breakfast and her second dose midafternoon—with no meals. I explained that the medication needs to be taken with food and that she was most likely experiencing low blood sugar in the afternoon, which could explain why she usually felt bad at that time of day. I suggested that she take the second dose with her evening meal. After a couple of weeks, I followed up with Mrs. T and she was elated! She said she felt so much better and thanked me for giving her afternoons back.

Pretty simple, right? Conduct a medication therapy review, uncover a problem, and create a medication-related action plan. Just changing the time Mrs. T was taking her medication led to an improvement in her health outcomes. My documentation of the initial review allowed for a follow-up check-in, and I learned that Mrs. T's issue had been resolved by the change. This MTM outreach provided a beneficial service to Mrs. T, even though I am not one of her regular health-care providers.

Problems can also arise because of the inconsistent training provided for those who conduct MTM, which can be provided through insurance companies, doctors, nurses, technicians, pharmacists, and "others." We already know that deprescribing is not currently a focus of the health-care curriculum, and who exactly do insurance companies classify as "other"? Because there is no gold standard for deprescribing and because each individual presents unique needs, how thorough and consistent is this practice, in general?

Furthermore, many providers are unable to bill insurance for MTM, so how likely are patients to pay out of pocket for this type of medication review? Especially if many of them have never heard of an MTM and have no idea that they need one?

Insurance Industry and Prescribing Conflicts

Here is an interesting quote from Andy Lazris, a primary care physician, that may shed light on medication overload:

If I lower my patient's blood pressure (to the point where) they fall and break their hip, I still get paid. But if their blood pressure is above the target, I fail the guideline.[88]

This situation is, of course, concerning and possibly alarming. I have heard directly from physicians that if you do not meet insurance and treatment options guidelines, then a patient may think you have failed them or an insurance company may question why you are not following the guidelines more aggressively. I tell such doctors that documentation is key, especially if the patient has doubts about the doctor's advice regarding deprescribing. However, documentation may not affect the target that insurance companies hold in high regard for payment and contract purposes.

In one of my discussions with a physicians' group, many questions were asked about deprescribing and physicians' willingness to deprescribe, how frequently they deprescribe, and if they would deprescribe another physician's medications. Many have deprescribed, but most expressed reservations about deprescribing another physician's medications for a patient. One primary care doctor rather candidly stated that cardiologists prescribe so many medications and rarely seem to reduce them, following every cardiovascular treatment guideline no matter the age of the patient. Later in the session, a cardiologist spoke up and admitted there can be issues caused by prescribing medications per the guidelines but that the potential of malpractice increases if the guidelines are not strictly followed.

I can completely see where all these physicians are coming from. Many of them understand that overprescribing for patients can lead to bad outcomes, but they also feel the need to follow medication guidelines in order to meet insurance requirements and lessen the risk of malpractice claims. As noted in the quote from Dr. Lazris above, doctors are aware that if they treat the patient toward the guideline, they meet the insurance requirements but the patient could fall. These issues are real and are cause for concern. The best option is to share the decision-making process with the patient and caregivers, including describing pros and cons of medications. I have seen many times in patient records that a certain therapy has been reviewed with the patient, who decided not to take the medication.

Many patients decide to not take a medication to prevent blood clots if they learn that they are at a high risk of excessive bleeding, as determined by the "HAS BLED" score as determined with their doctor. HAS BLED is based on high blood pressure systolic reading, abnormal kidney and liver function, a history of stroke, a bleeding tendency or history of a major bleed, labile or uncontrolled INR, if a patient is elderly (older than 65), and the use of drugs such as aspirin,

NSAIDS, and alcohol.[89] (INR stands for international normalized ratio, a test to check if your blood clots appropriately.) If a patient's HAS BLED score is high, then it may be safer to not take a medication that can prevent clots. These difficult decisions can be a part of shared decision-making.

Fragmented Electronic Medical Records

Electronic records are common in the pharmacy, the physician's office, and the hospital. However, these systems are not necessarily integrated and, in fact, are usually not integrated, at least in the United States. That means doctors and pharmacists may be looking at different medication records, but the patients do not realize the discrepancy. For example, a doctor tells a patient to reduce a medication from two tablets daily to one tablet and changes the in-office records. But the doctor does not send in a new prescription to the pharmacy because it is not a new medicine. When the patient gets a refill, it comes with the old instructions for two tablets daily because the pharmacist's records do not integrate with the doctor's records.

Another area of concern occurs during transitions of care. One hospitalist may make a change to a patient's medications during a hospitalization, but at discharge a different hospitalist may continue medications that the patient was taking prior to the hospitalization. Furthermore, if patients are returning to long-term care, medications may be inadvertently continued if they are not officially discontinued.

There are many more scenarios and barriers that could be discussed in this chapter; however, I think it should be clear that many entities play a part in the culture of polypharmacy. This is not all bad news! Medications have helped us live longer and healthier. The good news is that the medication culture has gotten us to this critical point; the bad news is that there is a critical point. In part IV, we will look at how we move forward, take action, and avoid overmedication, polypharmacy, and geriatric syndromes related to these issues.

Overview of Part III: Why Is Deprescribing So Hard?

- Though it looks as if it should be easy, deprescribing is filled with barriers constructed by the patient, caregivers, health-care providers, and the health-care system.

- More and more health-care researchers and organizations are warning about the harms of polypharmacy and recommending methods and guidelines to help health-care providers undertake a deprescribing process.

- Many levels of teamwork are needed to successfully implement and execute deprescribing.

- Conversations about deprescribing are best if continued throughout the continuum of care.

- Minimal guidelines are available to determine when a medication may become inappropriate for a patient.

- A patient's health goals are an important factor in shared decision-making to deprescribe.

- When reviewing outcomes of deprescribing, "no change" may be considered a success.

- Brand-name extensions, auto-refills, and insurance industry guidelines can add to the hazards of polypharmacy and make deprescribing more difficult.

- Medication reviews and Medication Therapy Management (MTM) can have great results but are sometimes limited based on health conditions, number and cost of medications, as well as coverage for such services.

Although modern medicine plays a large role in helping us live longer and better, polypharmacy is harming too many people. There are encouraging signs that our modern health-care system is beginning to see the benefits of cultivating a culture of deprescribing in order to take full advantage of our helpful medical advances.

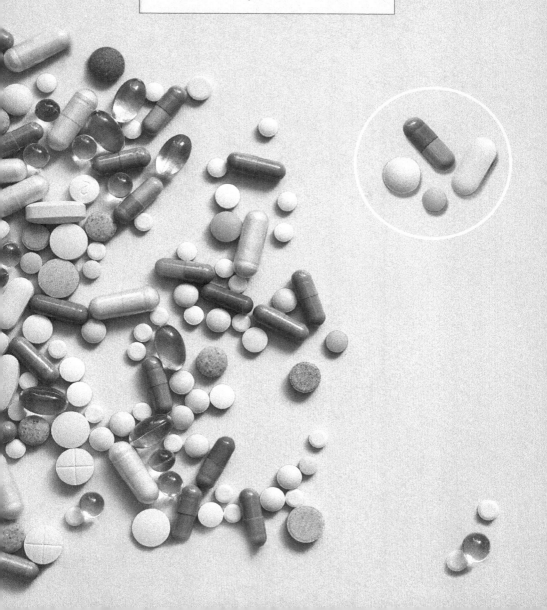

PART IV
The Way Forward

CHAPTER 11

Avoiding a MEDisaster

IN THE LATE 1800S SIR WILLIAM OSLER STATED, "The first duty of the physician is to educate the masses not to take medicine."[90] In his 2018 article "What Needs to Change to Make Deprescribing Doable," Dr. Ranit Mishori advocates for deprescribing to be taught along with prescribing in medical school.[91] Obviously a lot changed in medicine in the past couple of centuries. We developed some amazing medications to combat diseases that caused death and suffering for centuries, and we now expect to live longer, healthier lives because of our medications. But too much of a good thing can cause problems too, and now it's time to focus some of the attention of our health-care system on deprescribing to optimize, especially for older adults.

All of us—patients, caregivers, health-care providers, pharmacists, insurers, and anyone who plays a role in the health system—currently play a part in polypharmacy. Now it's time for all of us to play a part in the deprescribing process.

Let's first take a look at how we as patients play key roles in the rise of polypharmacy. How often do we expect to leave a doctor's office with a prescription? If we have an ache or illness, are we eager to consider a nonpharmacological approach to treatment? Are we willing to

- Change our diets to reduce stomach acid?
- Turn off our cell phones, tablets, and computers earlier in the evening to help us sleep better?
- Move more, walk more, reduce alcohol intake, or meditate to reduce blood pressure?
- Stop smoking or vaping to reduce lung and breathing issues?

How well do we understand the medications we are taking and their purpose? Or do we just take medications because we were "told to"? Are we overly influenced by the commercials we see for supplements and vitamins that promise to provide healthier joints, better cognition, cures for a low libido, and reversal of aging? As patients and health consumers, we expect products to make us feel better, work better, and improve our life. As a culture, we generally rely on products to keep us young and healthy.

However, we can be taking too much, combining too much, and even causing interactions and side effects that are viewed as a new problem and treated with another medication. We have so many places we can go to buy prescriptions, health products, and over-the-counter (OTC) formulations. We travel to various pharmacies for convenience or price. We use mail order, specialty pharmacies, and possibly compound pharmacies. We buy products online, at a supplement store, and through home-business / multi-level marketing sellers. We are provided products from well-meaning friends and family, who learned about them from television commercials and social media posts.

Providers and the basic infrastructure of the U.S. health-care system play roles in this polypharmacy culture as well. Most of us regularly visit several providers who have prescribing rights: primary doctors, specialists, hospitalists, nurse practitioners, physician assistants, dentists, opticians, ophthalmologists, and some pharmacists in a limited capacity. Do all these specialists take the time to determine everything you are taking, including prescription, OTC, and supplements? If a provider is prescribing something, do they check with the other specialists or change medications from the other providers?

How probable is it that the prescriber would call all your pharmacies and other providers to tell them you are no longer taking a medication? It is easy to see how medications can be added and not necessarily stopped. Health-care providers are well trained to treat and prescribe but probably not as well trained to reduce treatment or deprescribe.

Problems built into the system side include automatic refills that are not turned off when medications are stopped or changed and out-of-sync medical records. Can all your doctor's offices, pharmacies, and hospitals see your most recent medication record? You could be prescribed medications based on treatment guidelines that are not necessary and safe for your age or health condition. Is our health system set up for deprescribing? What type of education is available for those practicing to deprescribe?

We can see that we are all responsible for creating a culture that values deprescribing as well as prescribing. To do that, we need to be educated about the deprescribing process, work together, improve systems, and document changes in a universal manner.

IN REAL LIFE

The tale of two inhalers

Ms. F finds out at the pharmacy that a new inhaler she was prescribed for COPD needs a prior authorization from her insurer. (I think most people roll their eyes when they hear they need prior authorization, as it means they cannot get their prescription until the medication is approved by the insurance company. It can be a nuisance, but this type of formulary limitation is designed to reduce cost and improve safety, in some cases.) Ms. F really wants to start a medication right away to help control her COPD better. The pharmacist kindly calls her prescriber, who decides to prescribe another product that acts similarly, is in the same family of medicines, and is covered by Ms. F's insurance. The pharmacist fills the new prescription, and Ms. F goes home and starts to use it.

When Ms. F returns to the pharmacy in a few weeks to pick up other prescriptions, she discovers that the insurance has approved the original inhaler and it is waiting for her along with her other medications. She accepts the inhaler and begins to use it along with the alternative inhaler. Ms. F continues to use both and to get both prescriptions refilled.

During a hospital visit, Ms. F complains of very dry mouth and dry throat, and a medication review determines that she has been using both inhalers, a duplication of therapy. This duplicated family of inhalers can cause dry mouth and throat and make it difficult to swallow. The patient is counseled on the similarity of the medications, and one inhaler is deprescribed.

Ms. F's situation displays the involvement of multiple parties in the overmedication, polypharmacy "train ride." The prescriber, pharmacy, patient, and health system are all involved and responsible for this duplication.

The Good News

So where is the good news? The good news is that more and more people at all levels of our health-care system are starting to recognize the problems of polypharmacy and the benefits of deprescribing to optimize. Even many older adults who have been traditionally very resistant to changes in their medications say they are willing to take less if a prescriber makes that recommendation.[92] And more and more health-care providers, pharmacists, and insurers are beginning to understand the benefits that can come with deprescribing, especially for older adults.

Retiring our meds

Think about the number of years you work before retirement, maybe 30, 40, 50 years. I am sure many of you began working at a young age, and you may have loved the job you had when you were 25. But as you get older, your priorities and ambitions—and stamina—change. What was fun and exciting at 25 is not as interesting when you are 55 or 65 or 75, and at some point, the idea of retirement begins to beckon.

Some of us take medications for that long too. Perhaps a medication has worked well for you for years, maybe 30, 40, even 50 years. But it's still likely that a time will come when a medication needs to be retired. Maybe it has done its job, or our body has changed and it is no longer needed, or we need to take a safer alternative to keep us healthy. When we start to think about retirement, we may start thinking about what we want to change, such as moving to a warmer climate or learning something new. The same can be true for the medicines we take; we should be proactive so that we can remain healthy and active.

Retooling our system

Researchers have shown that educating health-care providers about the perils of polypharmacy and the benefits of deprescribing can encourage them to reduce or revise medications for their older patients. A study conducted in Parma, Italy, showed that working with general providers to help them identify potentially inappropriate medications and provide alternatives proved to be helpful in reducing the number of inappropriate medications prescribed to patients 65 of age and older.[93] The group who received fewer medications was found to have a reduction in unplanned hospitalizations during a year-long intervention monitored by the researchers.

This study provides evidence that reducing potentially inappropriate medications can reduce hospitalizations. It also demonstrates that deprescribing is not necessarily a one-time practice and that continued intervention may reduce unplanned hospitalizations— or at the very least, prevent an increase. The study revealed that a significant savings in health dollars can be achieved by reducing unplanned hospitalizations.

If deprescribing can reduce hospitalizations, it can also reduce the cost of health care, which can be a benefit to individuals, insurers, governments, and more. Imagine the savings and health outcomes we can achieve if we begin to promote a culture of deprescribing to optimize our health.

Another culture change that could pay large dividends would be to authorize pharmacists to visit patients' homes for a medication review. Visiting nurses and physical therapists are common in home health care, especially after a hospitalization. Pharmacist reviews in a person's home can be effective in assisting patients and caregivers with establishing the most effective medication schedules and organization as well as potentially deprescribing. Unfortunately, it's not terribly common that these visits are covered by insurance and few people think about paying a pharmacist out of pocket for such a service. But making such visits a common part of home health care could bring benefits to individuals as well as our health-care infrastructure.

Choosing Wisely

The Choosing Wisely Campaign is an initiative of the American Board of Internal Medicine Foundation that tries to promote dialogue between health-care providers and patients to help them avoid unnecessary medical tests, medications, treatments, and procedures. Through Choosing Wisely, the American Society of Health-System Pharmacists recommends that providers conduct a comprehensive review of a patient's medications, including OTC, supplements, and herbal products, before adding or continuing prescriptions for a patient taking five or more prescription medications.[94] The

American Geriatrics Society recommends providers not prescribe any medication without undertaking a drug review. These medication management recommendations can be rather time-consuming, which may be a barrier to some patients and prescribers, but evidence for the benefits of such an approach continue to mount.

Although these recommendations are aimed at providers, patients should also be aware of them. If your doctor recommends adding another prescription, start asking questions, especially if they have not conducted a full medication review. You can question the need of another medication, ask whether it will interact negatively with your other medications, and ask if you can stop taking any of your current prescriptions. This process allows for shared decision-making and open communication. Use the MedStrong Medication List and the MedStrong Question List provided in this book to help facilitate the process.

Remaining Vigilant

Years ago a friend and I were making plans to meet up together with our families. We were considering two different spots depending upon timing and our other commitments, and we considered canceling because we were not sure we could make it work out. But we texted back and forth and finally decided to meet. We each arrived at our destination at the time we had decided. Unfortunately, we were in two different places! We had never fully decided between our two meeting options, and she went one place and I went the other. Our children could not believe that the two of us were "that bad" at making plans via text.

Communication breakdowns can easily occur in everyday conversations, and texts and social media bring in new ways to misunderstand each other. Electronic prescribing is no different from any other type of digital communication. It's easy for one party or another to misinterpret information and hard to ensure that expected actions have been taken. When a doctor recommends deprescribing a medication, is that prescription canceled at the patient's pharmacy? Placed on hold? Maybe it has already been automatically refilled and is waiting in a bin for pick-up or en route to the patient by mail. Will the patient remember not to take the medication if it arrives in thier mailbox or is handed to them by the pharmacist? Or will the patient assume the delivery means the physician would like them to restart the medication?

I have spoken with physicians who feel automatic refills can have a negative impact on attempts to deprescribe. Possible drug duplication can occur when medications are changed to another strength or switched to another formulation, because all variations of the medications are auto-refilled and the patient may end up taking duplicates.

Some prescribers may speak only to the patient and caregivers regarding discontinuing medications but may not communicate directly with the pharmacy. Patients may neglect to tell the pharmacy about the discontinued medication and then call and ask "for all my prescriptions to be filled that can be filled," not knowing the pharmacy prescription records still list the "discontinued" medications unknowingly. Asking for "all my prescriptions" may also lead a pharmacy to provide older strengths or formulations of medications, which can cause overdosing or underdosing.

In other words, health-care providers, pharmacists, and individuals need to stay vigilant regarding medications. Keep the lines of communication open and be ready to ask questions and verify information no matter your role when prescribing, dispensing, taking, verifying, documenting, or reviewing medications.

As the Pendulum Swings

Humans are prone to "go all in," and "take it to the max." We encourage each other to "go big or go home." Patience may be a virtue, but we never hear sports fans yelling, "Patience! Patience!" as they cheer on their teams. We like to see immediate results and exceed all of our desired goals. Only in golf do you strive to be subpar!

But we should not approach deprescribing with an all-or-nothing mind-set. We do not want to swing the pendulum from polypharmacy to undertreatment. (See figure 11.1.) We know how dangerous medical pendulum swings can be because we recently witnessed one: when health-care providers began to perceive that pain was under-treated, we swung the pendulum so hard that we mired ourselves in a deadly opioid crisis. We need to settle into the sweet spot—the fulcrum of medication balance—as we try to move away from a culture of polypharmacy. It is so important to remember that deprescribing does not mean eliminating all medications or that most medications are no longer needed.

Deprescribing is not all or nothing. It's a process, a methodology that should be individualized. Deprescribing to optimize takes time, follow-through, and monitoring. Sometimes it might even require a restart to get it right.

Figure 11.1

Prescribing Pendulum

Under-medicated   **Over-medicated**

Optimal prescribing

Take Action!

We grew up learning "a stitch in time saves nine," that successful businesses are proactive instead of reactive, and that fixing something earlier rather than later can save a lot of money and disruption. Let's take the same approach with our bodies! Medications can be needed to treat health conditions or to prevent further progression of a health condition. But medications can sometimes cause problems, too, and may eventually need to be stopped or reduced or changed. A proactive approach to deprescribing can prevent falls, accidents, and hospitalizations.

Individuals should get started now making a MedStrong Medication Optimization Plan (MOP), using the many resources provided in earlier chapters and in the Resources section of this book. Providers should consider deprescribing before a patient suffers a fall or accident or debilitating side effect.

Every encounter between a patient and health-care provider is an opportunity to reduce unnecessary medications.[95]

That statement is probably my favorite takeaway from my research into deprescribing, and I hope that deprescribing soon becomes as much a part of our health-care culture as prescribing is now. Several steps are considered routine parts of meeting with a health-care provider today. During physicals you are asked about falling, wearing seat belts, and a host of other questions. Weight, height, and vitals are taken. Reviewing medications for need, safety, outcomes, and possible side effects should become routine practices too.

Now is the time to take action!

Become part of the cultural shift to deprescribe.

Be empowered to start the conversation.

Be MedStrong: Deprescribe to Optimize. DO!

Overview of Part IV: The Way Forward

- Patients, caregivers, health-care providers, and pharmacists all play a role in polypharmacy, and all can play a role in fostering a culture of deprescribing to optimize medications.
- The Choosing Wisely Campaign can help patients avoid unnecessary medications.
- As deprescribing begins to be more accepted, we all have to work to make sure the pendulum does not swing too far toward undermedicating patients.
- The MedStrong Optimization Plan (MOP) and the variety of checklists and forms in this book can help patients and providers begin a deprescribing process.

It's time for patients, caregivers, health-care providers, pharmacists, and every part of the health-care infrastructure to take action against the hazards of polypharmacy and begin deprescribing to optimize for health and well-being.

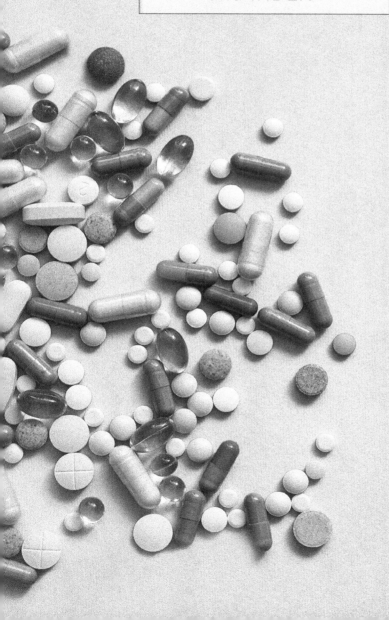

APPENDICES
and INDEX

Appendix A

MedStrong Medication Optimization Plan

Use the MedStrong MOP action guide and the question and decision lists provided in this section to help take action to tame your medications and determine if deprescribing to optimize is the right move for you now. You can make copies of these lists so that you can keep them updated and share them with each of your health-care providers and pharmacists.

MedStrong Medication Optimization Plan (MOP)
Step-by-Step Deprescribing Guide for the Patient

STEP 1
List all medications.
Fill out the MedStrong Medication List.

STEP 2
Review medication list.
Use the MedStrong Medication List and the MedStrong Question List to formulate questions.

STEP 3
Decide to deprescribe with your provider.
Start the "DO" conversation using the Medstrong Question List.

STEP 4
Make a plan.
Fill out the MedStrong Deprescribing Form.

STEP 5
Monitor, document, follow up.
Use the Medstrong Deprescribing Form and the MedStrong Medication Change Form.

MedStrong Medication List —Prescriptions

PRESCRIPTION Name of Prescription Medication and Strength of Dose	How Taken	Reason for Taking	Does the Problem Still Exist?	Is the Medical Condition Controlled?

MedStrong Medication List —Over-the-Counter (OTC)

OVER THE COUNTER OTC Medication, Supplement, or Herbal and Strength of Dose	How Taken	Reason for Taking	Does the Problem Still Exist?	Is the Medical Condition Controlled?

MedStrong Medication List Notes

Be truthful when making your list! Do you take more or less than what has been prescribed?

✔ Then list what you actually take, not what your doctor thinks you're taking.

✔ Write question marks where you are uncertain of the response.

When you are thinking about what nonprescription medicines you have taken, ask yourself these questions.

✔ Have I self-treated any ailments with nonprescription medications since my last medical visit?

✔ What problems? What did I use?

What Problem?	What I Used.

MedStrong Anticholinergic Burden Scoring Sheet

Date: _____   Scale Used: _____

Medication	Listed on Anticholinergic Scale? Y/N	Score
	Number of Medications Y =	Total:

Here is one of the calculators available online:
http://www.acbcalc.com

MedStrong Question List

Check the questions that fit your concerns to ask your health-care providers.

Questions to Ask Yourself

☐ Am I having problems paying for all of my prescriptions?

☐ Do I sometimes choose which medicines to take or not take because of affordability issues?

☐ Do I take some or all of my medications differently than how they were prescribed to "stretch them out"? For example, do I take a pill every other day even if it is prescribed to take daily?

Questions to Ask Your Health-Care Provider

☐ Are there any medications that I am currently taking that may no longer be necessary?

☐ Are there any medications that may be dosed too high for my age, health status, kidney function or with other medications I am taking?

☐ Could one of my health concerns actually be a side effect to a medication?

☐ Are there safer medications I could be taking?

☐ Can any of my medications increase my risk of falls?

☐ Can any combination of these medications increase my risk of falls or increase a risk of bleeding?

Questions to Ask at the Pharmacy

☐ Could I be using an OTC product to treat a side effect for one of my prescription medications?

☐ Is this OTC product okay to take with my current medications and my health conditions?

☐ Are any of my medications potentially being prescribed for a side effect of another prescription (prescribing cascade)?

☐ Could any of my medications increase my risk of falling? If so, which ones?

☐ If I could take fewer medications, which ones should I ask my doctor about possibly stopping?

☐ Am I taking any unnecessary medications?

☐ How long will it take for this medication to start working as it should?

☐ Is this a medication that I need to fill regularly?

☐ When would be the best time of day to take this medication?

☐ Is it possible for you to help me figure out a schedule to take my medications?

Questions to Ask When an Older Adult Is Hospitalized

☐ Could any of my medications—prescription, OTC, herbal, or supplements—have contributed to this condition?

☐ Could my medications have interacted to have caused my hospitalization, such as medications that have additive effects/side effects?

☐ Are there any of my current medications that might be unnecessary or that you think we should discuss with the primary care physician or specialist?

☐ Are there any medications, OTCs, supplements, that may be interacting with blood tests or any other tests or procedures?

Questions to Ask When Being Discharged From the Hospital

☐ Are there changes to my medications or how I should take them?

☐ Are there medications that are similar to medications that I take at home? I do not want to duplicate my medications.

☐ Are there any medications I should no longer take?

☐ How long should I continue taking any new medications? Are some just for a short period of time or just when needed?

My Questions about Specific Concerns or Specific Medications

_____

_____

_____

_____

_____

_____

_____

_____

_____

_____

_____

_____

_____

MedStrong Deprescribing Form

Medication: _____ Date: _____

Why is this medication being deprescribed? _____

Deprescribe Instructions: _____

☐ Changed to: _____

☐ Reduced to: _____

☐ Stopped: Date: _____

Taper: Yes ☐ No ☐

If yes, taper instructions: _____

_____

Monitor: _____

☐ Labs: _____ Date: _____

☐ Check: _____ and keep a log.

(Examples: blood pressure, heart rate, blood glucose, weight)

Date: _____ Time: _____ Results: _____

How do I feel?:

☐ No different: _____

☐ Not so good because: _____

☐ Better, I notice that: _____

Follow-up with:

Name of health care provider: _____

Phone number: _____

Date of next appointment: _____

MedStrong Medication Change Form

Medication and Strength	How Many, How Often	Prescribed by	Date/Year Started	Still Taking?	Date Medication Stopped or Changed	Medication Restarted or Changed, Why?

MedStrong Annual Physical Medication Checklist

My Medication and Strength	How Taken & When	Reason for the Medication	ACTION - Check the Box That Applies	
			Deprescribe	Continue

Appendix B
Medication List

Class/Family of Medication	Generic Names
Anticholinergics used for	
urinary incontinence	oxybutynin, solifenacin, tolterodine
COPD	aclidinium, ipratropium, tiotropium, umeclidinium
parkinsonism	parkinsonism benztropine
stomach spasm	dicyclomine, hyoscyamine
motion sickness, nausea, vomiting	scopolamine
Antidepressants	
SSRIs	fluoxetine, paroxetine, sertraline, citalopram, escitalopram
SNRIs	duloxetine, venlafaxine
TCAs	amitriptyline, nortriptyline
Others	bupropion, mirtazapine, trazodone
Antihistamines	
First Generation	brompheniramine, chlorpheniramine, clemastine, diphenhydramine, doxylamine, meclizine
Second Generation	cetirizine, fexofenadine, loratadine
Antipsychotics	
Second Generation	aripiprazole, clozapine, iloperidone, lurasidone, olanzapine, paliperidone, pimavanserin, quetiapine, risperidone, ziprasidone
First Generation	haloperidol
Antiseizure	
Hydantoin	phenytoin
Miscellaneous	carbamazepine, lamotrigine, levetiracetam, oxcarbazepine, topiramate, valproic acid, zonisamide

Class/Family of Medication   Generic Names

Benzodiazepines	
alprazolam, clonazepam, diazepam, lorazepam, oxazepam, temazepam, triazolam	

Bisphosphonates	
alendronate, ibandronate, risedronate	

Blood Pressure Medications	
ACE inhibitors	benazepril, captopril, enalapril, lisinopril, quinapril
ARBs	losartan, olmesartan, valsartan
Beta-blockers	atenolol, metoprolol, nebivolol
Calcium channel blockers	amlodipine, diltiazem, verapamil
Diuretics: Loop	bumetanide, ethacrynic acid, furosemide, torsemide
Potassium-sparing	amiloride, eplerenone, spironolactone, triamterene
Thiazide	chlorthalidone, hydrochlorothiazide

Dementia Medications	
Acetylcholinesterase inhibitors	donepezil, galantamine, rivastigmine
NMDA receptor antagonist	memantine

Diabetes Medications	
Biguanide	metformin
DDP-4 inhibitors	linagliptin, saxagliptin, sitagliptin
Insulin	insulin-aspart, -degludec, -detemir, -glargine, -lispro, -NPH, regular
Meglitinide	nateglinide, repaglinide
SGLT2 inhibitor	canagliflozin, dapagliflozin, empagliflozin
Sulfonylureas	glipizide, glyburide, glimepiride
Thiazolidinedione	pioglitazone, rosiglitazone

Class/Family of Medication	Generic Names
Eyedrops for Glaucoma	
Carbonic anhydrase inhibitors	brinzolamide, dorzolamide
Beta blocker	timolol
Prostaglandin analog	bimatoprost, latanoprost, travoprost

GABA analog
Gabapentin, pregabalin

NSAIDs
diclofenac, ibuprofen, naproxen, meloxicam

Proton Pump Inhibitors (PPIs)
dexlansoprazole, esomeprazole, lansoprazole, omeprazole, pantoprazole, rabeprazole

Statins
atorvastatin, fluvastatin, lovastatin, pitavastatin, pravastatin, rosuvastatin, simvastatin

Glossary

Absorption: The ability of medicine to transfer from the gut to the bloodstream.

ACE inhibitors (angiotensin-converting enzyme inhibitors): A family of medicine used to treat high blood pressure.

Adverse drug event: A harmful outcome to a medication.

Agent: Another word for medication or drug.

Anticholinergics: Medications that are used to treat urinary incontinence. These medications can cause very drying effects. Other medications also have anticholinergic side effects, which can cause fast heart rate, cognition changes, and increased risk of falls.

Antiplatelet medications: A family of medicines that reduce the effects of platelets to reduce the risk of blood clots.

ARBs (Angiotensin II receptor blockers): A family of medicines used to treat high blood pressure. Examples include: losartan, valsartan, irbesartan, candesartan.

Benzodiazepines: A family of medicines used for anxiety. Examples are lorazepam, oxazepam, triazolam, alprazolam, clonazepam.

Bisphosphonates: A family of medications used to treat osteoporosis (brittle bones).

Chronic disease: A health condition that one lives with and potentially treats to reduce worsening of condition overtime or to reduce symptoms of the condition over time.

Citalopram: A medication used to treat depression and anxiety.

Clinical inertia: Knowing there is a potential problem but not knowing how or when to take action such as deprescribing.

Cognitive bias: Thinking more subjectively, based on one's experience, than objectively, around the current circumstances or situation.

Comorbidity: More than one health condition that a person may have.

COPD (chronic obstructive pulmonary disease): Lung condition that causes difficulty with breathing, often due to smoking and other irritant exposure or chronic asthma.

COX-2-Inhibitor: A family of medications that is used for pain and inflammation. An example is celecoxib.

Culture of health care: The behaviors and expectations that society has regarding the practice of health care.

Deprescribing: The act or process of thoughtfully reducing, switching, or stopping medications that may be inappropriate or no longer necessary.

Diphenhydramine: An over-the-counter antihistamine medication used to treat allergies and allergic reactions. It is also used in cough and cold medications and in medications to help one sleep.

Distribution: The pathway of a drug throughout the body systems.

Diuretic: A type of medication used to eliminate fluid, sometimes called a "water pill." Can be used for edema (such as swollen ankles), high blood pressure, and heart failure.

Drug-disease interaction: When a medication causes another health condition to worsen.

Drug-drug interaction: When one or more medications cause another medication to not work as expected.

Drug-food interaction: When a medication interferes with the expected outcome of a medication.

Elimination: The removal of a drug from the body through urine and feces.

Falls: The unintentional act of landing on the ground.

Formulary: List of medications covered by an insurance company or available at a facility such as a hospital.

Gabapentin: Medication that was originally used to treat seizures and is more commonly used for nerve-type pain, including neuropathy.

Glipizide: A medication used to treat diabetes.

Glyburide: A medication used to treat diabetes.

HbA1c: A blood test that determines the average blood sugar over 3 months.

Heart failure: A health condition where the heart is unable to pump blood as well or fill as well. There are many stages of this condition.

High-risk medications: Medications that have an increased chance of becoming toxic and causing harm instead of benefit.

Hydrochlorothiazide (HCTZ): A type of diuretic ("water pill").

Hypoglycemia: Low blood sugar.

Indication: The condition that a medication is being used for.

Isosorbide: A type of medication in the nitrate family used for angina; there are two forms: isosorbide dinitrate and isosorbide mononitrate.

Medication therapy management (MTM): A step-by-step process of reviewing a patient's medications, identifying possible medication-related problems, and determining an action plan to reduce problems.

Metabolism: The chemical changes of a medication within the body necessary to activate the medication and/or make it so that the medication can be eliminated.

NSAIDs (nonsteroidal anti-inflammatory drugs): A family of medicines used to treat pain and inflammation. Examples are ibuprofen, naproxen, diclofenac, indomethacin.

Optimize: To maximize benefit and reduce harm with the least amount of medications, with the lowest appropriate dose, at the correct frequency, while monitoring for appropriate and best outcomes.

Orthostatic hypotension: A drop in blood pressure when changing position—for example, sitting to standing.

Overmedication: The excessive or inappropriate use or continuation of unnecessary medication.

Pharmacodynamics: What the drug does to a body, its actions and side effects.

Pharmacokinetics: What the body does to a drug: absorption, distribution, metabolism, and elimination.

Polypharmacy: Multiple medications, typically five or more, that a person takes.

Potentially inappropriate medications: Medications that pose more harm then benefit or may be unnecessary.

Potentially inappropriate prescribing: Prescribing of high-risk medications, unnecessary medications, or medications to treat a side effect rather than addressing the problem-causing drug, when another, safer option may be used.

Prescribing-cascade: The use of medication to treat the side effects of another medication.

Proton pump inhibitors (PPI): Medications used to treat stomach acid problems such as GERD, or gastric esophageal reflux disorder.

Readmission: Having to be hospitalized again soon after being discharged from a hospital, typically within 30 days.

Shared decision-making: When patient and prescribers discuss patient goals and therapy goals and reach a decision on treatment (or nontreatment) of a condition together.

Simvastatin: A medication used to treat cholesterol.

Statins: A family of medicines used to treat high cholesterol. Examples are atorvastatin, simvastatin, rosuvastatin.

Telehealth: A way in which health-care professionals can communicate long-distance with a patient, typically via the phone or computer audio and video.

Tramadol: A medication in the opioid family that is used for pain.

Transitions of care: A shift in responsibility of care for an individual from place to place; for example from hospital to home.

Treatment guidelines: An algorithm to treat a health condition grounded in evidence-based medicine and decided upon through a panel of experts.

Z-drugs: A family of medicines used as sleep aids. Examples include zolpidem, zopiclone, eszopiclone, zaleplon.

Zolpidem: A medication used to treat insomnia.

Resources

American Geriatrics Society (AGS)
(https://www.americangeriatrics.org)
(https://www.americangeriatrics.org/publications-tools/
patient-education)
The home of The Beers Criteria, which highlight medications that
could be potentially inappropriate in patients.

American Geriatrics Society's Health in Aging Foundation
(www.Healthinaging.org)
The Health in Aging website offers a number of information
sheets for the health-care consumer to view, including "Ten
Medications Older Adults Should Avoid or Use with Caution."

**American Society of Consultant Pharmacists (ASCP)
Foundation** (https://www.ascp.com/page/foundation) and
**American Society of Consultant Pharmacists (ASCP)
Foundation** (https://www.ascp.com)
provides a website called Help With My Meds (helpwithmymeds.
org) (https://www.ascp.com/mpage/Care_Pharmacist) that can
help users find a senior-care pharmacist in your area. Board-
certified geriatric pharmacists are available in every state, Canada,
and Australia.

Anticholinergic Burden Calculator (http://www.acbcalc.com)
This calculator helps to calculate and find a score for medications
that can cause anticholinergic effects, including dry effects, confusion, fast heartbeat, and falls.

Chronic Heart Failure Action Plan (https://assets.heartfoundation.
org.nz/documents/shop/heart-healthcare/non-stock-resources/heart-
failure-action-plan.pdf)
My Heart Failure Action Plan by Heart Foundation provides a daily
check-in and action guide to monitor heart failure to help maintain
a better quality of life and prevent hospitalization.

Chronic Obstructive Pulmonary Disease (COPD) Action Plan
(https://www.lung.org/getmedia/c7657648-a30f-4465-af92-
fc762411922e/fy20-ala-copd-action-plan.pdf)
My COPD Action Plan by the American Lung Association provides
a daily check-in and action guide to monitor COPD to help maintain
a better quality of life and prevent hospitalization.

Choosing Wisely (https://www.choosingwisely.org/societies/
american-geriatrics-society/)
Choosing Wisely, a program offered through the American Board
of Internal Medicine, highlights several concerns that we should
heed as health-care consumers. Though it is intended to be a guide
for prescribers, individuals can review it to help start conversations
with providers.

Clinical Frailty Scale (https://www.dal.ca/sites/gmr/our-tools/clini-
cal-frailty-scale.html)
This scale shows varying levels of frailty from very fit to end of life.
Challenge yourself to move up the scale for better quality of life and
health.

The Comprehensive Geriatric Assessment
(https://www.cgakit.com/cga)
Assessment toolkits for health-care professionals to assess and evaluate older adults on quality of life, mobility, and fall prevention.

Deprescribing.org
This Canadian program is actively reviewing deprescribing. The
organization has begun to review and provide algorithms to deprescribe or reduce medications such as benzodiazepines, proton pump
inhibitors, antiseizure medications, and antidiabetic medications.

Drive to Deprescribe (https://paltc.org/drive2deprescribe)
Programming available for facilities and health-care professionals to
institute education and goals of reducing and optimizing medications
in post-acute and long-term care settings.

Drugs.com
Website available for learning about medications (both prescription
and nonprescription), checking potential drug interactions, and
identifying pills.

Lown Institute (https://lowninstitute.org/reports/medication-over-load-americas-other-drug-problem/)
Lown Institute is a think tank that advocates for a "just and caring system for health." The publications are thorough and provide great ideas, examples, and statistics.

Medstopper (http://medstopper.com)
This website can help identify potentially inappropriate medications and the priority in which one may want to consider deprescribing medication.

Mini Mental Status Examination (MMSE)
(https://www.dementiacarecentral.com/mini-mental-state-exam/)
This website provides the MMSE along with a host of information for people caring for those with dementia.

STOPPFall (Screening Tool of Older Persons Prescriptions in older adults with high fall risk) (https://academic.oup.com/ageing/article/50/4/1189/6043386)
This tool considers whether withdrawal of a medication should be considered for potential adverse events, especially if a person is at a high risk of falls.

Stopping Elderly Accidents, Deaths, and Injuries (STEADI)
(https://www.cdc.gov/steadi/index.html)
This program from the Centers for Disease Control (CDC) aims to help prevent falls. It educates individuals and health-care professionals about screening for and preventing falls, accidents, and injuries that can lead to death in older adults. There are many options to choose from for information on preventing falls, including SAFE:
- Screen for medications that could increase falls, injury, accidents;
- Assess for the best treatment for the individual's active health conditions;
- Formulate an action plan to optimize treatment; and
- Educate the individual and caregiver on medication changes and reducing falls, accidents, and injuries.

WISE & WELL Dr. Donna Bartlett (https://donnabartlett.com)
This website is dedicated to learning more about deprescribing and to share deprescribing stories.

Endnotes

1. Rankin A, Cadogan CA, Patterson SM, et al. Interventions to improve the appropriate use of polypharmacy for older people. *Cochrane Database Syst Rev.* 2018;(9):CD008165.

2. Reeve E, Gnjidic D, Long J, Hilmer S. A systematic review of the emerging definition of 'deprescribing' with network analysis: implications for future research and clinical practice. *Br J Clin Pharmacol.* 2015;80(6):1254–1268. doi:10.1111/bcp.1273

3. Scott IA, Gray LC, Martin JH, et al. Deciding when to stop: towards evidence-based deprescribing of drugs in older adults. *Evid Based Med.* 2013;18(4):121–124.

4. Hajjar ER, Gray SL, Slattum PW, et al. Geriatrics. In *Pharmacotherapy: A Pathophysiological Approach.* 9th ed. McGraw-Hill Education, 2014.

5. Hajjar ER, Hanlon JT. Polypharmacy in elderly patients. *Am J Geriatr Pharmacother.* 2007;5(4):345–351.

6. National Institute on Alcohol Abuse and Alcoholism. Harmful interactions: mixing alcohol with medicines. Updated November 2020. Accessed March 10, 2022. https://www.niaaa.nih.gov/sites/default/files/publications/NIAAA_Harmful_Interactions_English.pdf

7. McGrath K, Hajjar ER, Kumar C, Hwang C, Salzman B. Deprescribing: a simple method for reducing polypharmacy. *J Fam Pract.* 2017;66(7):436–445.

8. Huizer-Pajkos A, Kane AE, Howlett SE, et al. Adverse geriatric outcomes secondary to polypharmacy in a mouse model: the influence of aging. *J Gerontol Ser A Biol Sci Med Sci.* 2016;71:571–577.

9. Potter K, Flicker L, Page A, Etherton-Beer C. Deprescribing in frail older people: a randomized controlled trial. PLOS ONE. 2016;1–21.doi: 10.1371/journal.pone.0149984

10. Brookes L. Easy to start, hard to stop: polypharmacy and deprescribing. *Medscape*. Jun 1, 2017.

11. Jansen J, Naganathan V, Carter SM, et al. Too much medicine in older people? Deprescribing through shared decision making. *BMJ*. 2016;353:i2893.

12. Farrell B, Mangin D. Deprescribing is an essential part of good prescribing. *Am Fam Physician*. 2019;99(1):7–9.

13. By the 2019 American Geriatrics Society Beers Criteria® Update Expert Panel. American Geriatrics Society 2019 Updated AGS Beers Criteria® for Potentially Inappropriate Medication Use in Older Adults. *J Am Geriatr Soc*. 2019;67(4):674–694.

14. O'Mahony DO, O'Sullivan D, Byrne S, et al. STOPP/START criteria for potentially inappropriate prescribing in older people: version 2. *Age Ageing*. 2015;44(2):213–218. doi:10.1093/ageing/afu145

15. Seppala LJ, Petrovic M, Ryg J, et al. STOPPFall (Screening Tool of Older Persons Prescriptions in older adults with high fall risk):a Delphi study by the EuGMS Task and Finish Group on fall-risk-increasing drugs. *Age Ageing*. 2020;1–11. doi:10.1093/ageing/afaa249

16. Liew TM, Lee CS, Liang Gob SK, Chang ZY. Potentially inappropriate prescribing among older persons: a meta-analysis of observational studies. *Ann Fam Med*. 2019;17(3):257–266.

17. Seppala LJ, Petrovic M, Ryg J, et al. STOPPFall (Screening Tool of Older Persons Prescriptions in older adults with high fall risk):a Delphi study by the EuGMS Task and Finish Group on fall-risk-increasing drugs. *Age Ageing*. 2020;1–11. doi:10.1093/ageing/afaa249

18. Maher RL, Hanlon J, Hajjar ER. Clinical consequences of polypharmacy in elderly. *Expert Opin Drug Saf*. 2014;13(1):57–65. doi:10.1517/14740338.2013.827660

19. Jyrkkä J, Enlund H, Lavikainen P, Sulkava R, Hartikainen S. Association of polypharmacy with nutritional status, functional ability and cognitive capacity over a three-year period in an

elderly population. *Pharmacoepidemiol Drug Saf.* 2011;20(5):514–522. doi:10.1002/pds.2116. Epub 2011 Feb 9. PMID: 21308855.

20. Heuberger RA, Caudell K. Polypharmacy and nutritional status in older adults: a cross-sectional study. *Drugs Aging.* 2011;28(4):315–23. doi:10.2165/11587670-000000000-00000 . PMID: 21428466.

21. Osson IN, Runnamo R, Engfeldt P. Medication quality and quality of life in the elderly, a cohort study. *Health Qual Life Outcomes.* 2011;9:95.

22. Scott IA, Hilmer SN, Reeve E, et al. Reducing inappropriate polypharmacy: the process of deprescribing. *JAMA Inter Med.* 2015;175(5):827–834.

23. Woodward MC. Deprescribing: achieving better health outcomes for older people through reducing medications. *J Pharm Pract Res.* 2003;33:323–328.

24. Reeve E, Thompson W, Farrell B. Deprescribing: a narrative review of the evidence and practical recommendations for recognizing opportunities and taking action. *Eur J Intern Med.* 2017;38:3–11.

25. Farrell B, Mangin D. Deprescribing is an essential part of good prescribing. *Am Fam Physician.* 2019;99(1):7–9.

26. Duncan P, Duerden M, Payne RA. Deprescribing: a primary care perspective. *Eur J Hosp Pharm.* 2017;24:37–42.

27. Scott IA, Hilmer SN, Reeve E, et al. Reducing inappropriate polypharmacy: the process of deprescribing. *JAMA Inter Med.* 2015;175(5):827–834.

28. Iyer S, Naganathan V, McLachlan AL, Le Couteur DG. Medication withdrawal trials in people age 65 years and older: a systematic review. *Drugs Aging.* 2008;25(12)1021–1031.

29. Van der Cammen TJM, Rajkumar C, Onder G, et al. Drug cessation in complex older adults: time for action. *Age Ageing.* 2014;43(1):20–25.

30. Tannenbaum C, Martin P, Tamblyn R, et al. Reduction of inappropriate benzodiazepine prescriptions among older adults through direct patient education: the EMPOWER cluster randomized trial. *JAMA Intern Med.* 2014;174(6):890–898.

31. American Heart Association Scientific Sessions 2020, Presentation MP269. Black patients less likely to receive added, higher dose meds to control blood pressure. *Newsroom.* November 9, 2020. https://newsroom.heart.org/news/black-patients-less-likely-to-receive-added-higher-dose-meds-to-control-blood-pressure

32. Reeve E, Wiese MD, Hendrix I, et al. People's attitudes, beliefs, and experiences regarding polypharmacy and willingness to deprescribe. *JAGS.* 2013;61(9):1508–1514.

33. McGrath K, Hajjar ER, Kumar C, Hwang C, Salzman B. Deprescribing: a simple method for reducing polypharmacy. *J Fam Pract.* 2017;66(7):436–445.

34. Farrell B, Mangin D. Deprescribing is an essential part of good prescribing. *American Family Physician.* 2019;99(1):7–9.

35. Brody JE. The risks of the prescribing cascade. *NY Times.* September 7, 2020, updated September 10, 2020.

36. Duncan P, Duerden M, Payne RA. Deprescribing: a primary care perspective. *Eur J Hosp Pharm.* 2017;24:37–42.

37. Royal Pharmaceutical Society. Medicines Optimisation. Helping patients to make the most of medicines. 2013. https://www.rpharms.com/Portals/0/RPS%20document%20library/Open%20access/Policy/helping-patients-make-the-most-of-their-medicines.pdf

38. Marvin V, Ward E, Poots AJ, Heard K, Rajagopalan A, Jubraj B. Deprescribing medicines in the acute setting to reduce the risk of falls. *Eur J Hosp Pharm.* 2017;24:10–15.

39. Tija J, Briesacher BA, Peterson D, et al. Use of medications of questionable benefit in advanced dementia. *JAMA Intern Med.* 2014. doi:10,1001/jamaintermed.2014.4103

40. Jansen J, Naganathan V, Carter SM, et al. Too much medicine in older people? Deprescribing through shared decision making. *BMJ*. 2016;353:i2893.

41. Philips LS, Branch WT, Cook CB, et al. Clinical inertia. *Ann Intern Med*. 2001;135:825–834.

42. Anderson K, Stowasser D, Freeman C, Scott I. Prescriber barriers and enablers to minimizing potentially inappropriate medications in adults: a systematic review and thematic synthesis. *BMJ Open*. 2014;4:e006544.

43. Hanlon P, Quinn TJ, Gallacher KI, et al. Assessing risks of polypharmacy involving medications with anticholinergic properties. *Ann Fam Medicine*. 2020;18(2):148–155.

44. Rice SD, Kim N, Farris C. Anticholinergic cognitive burden in older people over acute admission. *Sr Care Pharm*. 2021;36(2): 104–111.

45. Van Poelgeest EP, Pronk AC, Rhebergen D, van der Velde N. Depression, antidepressants and fall risk: therapeutic dilemmas-a clinical review. *Eur Geriatr Med*. 2021;12(3):585–596. doi:10.1007/s41999-021-00475-7

46. McGrath K, Hajjar ER, Kumar C, Hwang C, Salzman B. Deprescribing: a simple method for reducing polypharmacy. *J Family Pract*. 2017;66(7):436–445.

47. Tannenbaum C, Martin P, Tamblyn R, et al. Reduction of inappropriate benzodiazepine prescriptions among older adults through direct patient education: the EMPOWER cluster randomized trial. *JAMA Intern Med*. 2014;174 (6):890–898.

48. Brookes L. Deprescribing cholinesterase inhibitors and memantine in people with dementia. *Medscape*. 2018. https://www.medscape.com/viewarticle/893256

49. Rea F, Biffi A, Ronco R, et al. Cardiovascular outcomes and mortality associated with discontinuing statins in older patients receiving polypharmacy. *JAMA Network Open*. 2021;4(6):e2113186.

50. Giral P, et al. Cardiovascular effect of discontinuing statins for primary prevention at the age of 75 years: a nationwide population-based cohort study in France. *Eur Heart J.* 2019;40(43): 3516–3525.

51. Reeve E, Thompson W, Farrell B. Deprescribing: a narrative review of the evidence and practical recommendations for recognizing opportunities and taking action. *Eur J Intern Med.* 2017;38:3–11.

52. Parker B, Thompson P. Effect of statins on skeletal muscle: exercise, myopathy, and muscle outcomes. *Exerc Sport Sci Rev.* 2012;40(4):188–194.

53. Shetty V, Chowta MN, Chowta NK, et al. Evaluation of potential drug-drug interactions with medications prescribed to geriatric patients in a tertiary care hospital. *J of Aging Research.* 2018;5728957:1–6.

54. McGrath K, Hajjar ER, Kumar C, Hwang C, Salzman B. Deprescribing: a simple method for reducing polypharmacy. *J of Fam Pract.* 2017;66(7):436–445.

55. Li Y, Delcher C, Wei YJ, et al. Risk of opioid overdose associated with concomitant use of opioids and skeletal muscle relaxants: a population-based cohort study. *Clin Pharmacol & Ther.* 2020;108(1):81–89. doi:10.1002/cpt.1807

56. US Food and Drug Administration. FDA requires new warnings for gabapentinoids about risk of respiratory depression. FDA in Brief. December 19, 2019. https://www.fda.gov/news-events/fda-brief/fda-brief-fda-requires-new-warnings-gabapentinoids-about-risk-respiratory-depression

57. Gomes T, Juurlink DN, Antoniou T, et al. Gabapentin, opioids, and the risk of opioid-related death: a population-based nested case-control study. *PLOS Medicine.* October 3, 2017. doi:org/10.1371

58. Gavin K. Use of risky brain-affecting drug combinations rising among seniors. The Lab. (University of Michigan). February 14,

2017. https://labblog.uofmhealth.org/rounds/use-of-risky-brain-affecting-drug-combinations-rising-among-seniors

59. Glans M, Kragh Ekstam A, Jakobsson U, et al. Risk factors for hospital readmission in older adults within 30 days of discharge: a comparative retrospective study. *BMC Geriatr.* 2020;20:467. https://doi.org/10.1186/s12877-020-01867-3

60. Shull MT, Braitman LE, Stites SD, DeLuca A, Hauser D. Effects of a pharmacist-driven intervention program on hospital readmissions. *Am J Health Syst Pharm.* 2018;75(9):e221–e230. doi: 10.2146/ajhp170287. PMID: 29691265.

61. Hanlon JT, Schmader KE, Samsa GP, et al. A method for assessing drug therapy appropriateness. *J Clin Epidemiol.* 1992;45(10):1045–51. doi:10.1016/0895-4356(92)90144-c . PMID: 1474400.

62. Hanlon JT, Schmader KE. The medication appropriateness index at 20: where it started, where it has been, and where it may be going. *Drugs Aging.* 2013;30(11):893–900. doi:10.1007/s40266-013-0118-4 . PMID: 24062215; PMCID: PMC3831621.

63. Woodward M. Deprescribing: achieving better health outcomes for older people through reducing medications. *Pharm Pracr Res.* 2003;33:323–328.

64. Potter K, Page A, Clifford R, Etherton-Beer C. Deprescribing: a guide for medication reviews. *J Pharm Pract Res.* 2016;46:358–367. (Official Publication of The Society of Hospital Pharmacists of Australia).

65. Farrell B, Mangin D. Deprescribing is an essential part of good prescribing. *Am Fam Physician.* 2019;99(1):7–9.

66. Scott IA, Hilmer SN, Reeve E, et al. Reducing inappropriate polypharmacy: the process of deprescribing. *JAMA Inter med.* 2015;175(5):827–834.

67. Lai L, Fok M. Drug-related problems and deprescribing in older adults. *BCMJ.* 2017;59(3):178–184.

68. Brookes L. Deprescribing benzodiazepines: changing attitudes. *Medscape.* June 15, 2018. https://www.medscape.com/viewarticle/897919_1

69. Farrell B, Mangin D. Deprescribing is an essential part of good prescribing. *Am Fam Physician.* 2019;99(1):7–9.

70. Duraisingham S, Jubraj B, Marvin V, et al. Stopping inappropriate medicines in the outpatient setting. *GM.* 2015;(April):35–41.

71. Scott IA, Hilmer SN, Reeve E, et al. Reducing inappropriate polypharmacy: the process of deprescribing. *JAMA Inter Med.* 2015;175(5):827–834.

72. Reeve E, Shakib S, Hendrix I, et al. The benefits and harms of deprescribing. *MJA.* 2014;201(7):1–4.

73. Duraisingham S, Jubraj B, Marvin V, et al. Stopping inappropriate medicines in the outpatient setting. *GM.* 2015;(April):35–41.

74. Page A, Etherton-Beer C. Undiagnosing to prevent overprescribing. *Maturitas.* 2019;(123):67–72.

75. Page A, Etherton-Beer C. Undiagnosing to prevent overprescribing. *Maturitas.* 2019;123:67–72.

76. Farrell B, Richardson L, Raman-Wilms L, et al. Self-efficacy for deprescribing: A survey for health care professionals using evidence-based deprescribing guidelines. *Res Social Admin Pharm.* 2018;14:18–25.

77. Reeve E, Shakib S, Hendrix I, et al. The benefits and harms of deprescribing. *MJA.* 2014;201(7):1–4.

78. AlRasheed MM, Alhawassi TM, Alanazi N, et al. Knowledge and willingness of physicians about deprescribing among older patients: a qualitative study. *Clin Interv Aging.* 2018;13:1401–1408.

79. Masters PA. Undoing what we've done: why deprescribing is so difficult. KevinMD.com. May 8, 2018. https://www.kevinmd.com/2018/05/undoing-what-weve-done-why-deprescribing-is-so-difficult.html

80. Reeve E, Thompson W, Farrell B. Deprescribing: a narrative review of the evidence and practical recommendations for recognizing opportunities and taking action. *Eur J Intern Med.* 2017;38:3–11.

81. Bloomstone S, Anzuoni K, Cocoros N, et al. Prescribing cascades in persons with Alzheimer's disease: engaging patients, caregivers, and providers in a qualitative evaluation of print educational materials. *Ther Adv Drug Saf.* 2020;11:1–13.

82. Green AR, Boyd CB, Gleason KS, et al. Designing a primary care-based deprescribing intervention for patients with dementia and multiple chronic conditions. *J Gen Intern Med.* 2020;35(12):3556–3563.

83. Reeve E, Wolff JL, Skehan M, et al. Assessment of attitudes toward deprescribing in older Medicare beneficiaries in the United States. *JAMA Intern Med.* 2018;178(12):1673–1680. doi:10.1001/jamainternmed.2018.4720

84. Garber J, Brownlee S. Medication overload: America's other drug problem. Lown Institute. April 2019:1–51. https://lowninstitute. org/reports/medication-overload-americas-other-drug-problem/

85. McKeirnan KC, Frazier KR, Yabusaki AA. Unintentional diphenhydramine use leading to falls in an older adult. *Senior Care Pharmacist.* 2020;35(3):113–119.

86. Brown M. Medication management: save time by simplifying your prescribing and refill process. *AMA STEPSforward.* December 19, 2019. https://edhub.ama-assn.org/steps-forward/ module/2757863

87. American Pharmacists Association, National Association of Chain Drug Stores Foundation. *Medication therapy management in pharmacy practice: core elements of an MTM service model.* Version 2.0. 2008. https://aphanet.pharmacist.com/sites/ default/files/files/core_elements_of_an_mtm_practice.pdf

88. Garber J, Brownlee S. Medication overload: America's other drug problem. Lown Institute. April 2019:1–51.

89. Pisters R, Lane DA, Nieuwlaat R, et al. HAS-BLED Score for major bleeding risk. *Evidencio*. 2015–2022. v.3.9. https://www. evidencio.com/models/show/163

90. Bean RB. *Sir William Osler: Aphorisms from His Bedside Teachings & Writings*. New York: Henry Schuman, 1950.

91. Mishori R. What needs to change to make deprescribing doable. *Fam Pract Manag*. 2018;25(3):5–6.

92. Reeve E, Wolff JL, Skehan M, et al. Assessment of attitudes toward deprescribing in older Medicare beneficiaries in the United States. *JAMA Intern Med*. 2018;178(12):1673–1680.

93. Alcusky M, Thomas RB, Jafari N, et al. Reduction in unplanned hospitalizations associated with a physician focused intervention to reduce potentially inappropriate medication use among older adults: a population-based cohort study. *BMC Geriatrics*. 2021;21:218.

94. American Geriatrics Society. Ten things clinicians and patients should question. Choosing Wisely. February 21, 2013. Last reviewed 2021. https://www.choosingwisely.org/societies/ american-geriatrics-society

95. Brookes L. Deprescribing benzodiazepines: changing attitudes. *Medscape*. June 15, 2018. https://www.medscape.com/ viewarticle/897919_1

Index

U

uncertainty, 143–44

underprescribing, 31

underuse of medication, 12–13

urinary incontinence, 28–29, 86
    anticholinergics used for, 74

urinary tract infections (UTIs), 88

V

vitamin B12, 98

vitamin C, 98

vitamin D, 98

vomiting, 74
    anticholinergics used for, 74

W

warfarin, 121, 122–23

water pills. *See* diuretics

Z

Zantac, 153, 154

Zantac 360°, 153

Zizza, Anthony, 149

zolpidem, 108, **135**, 136

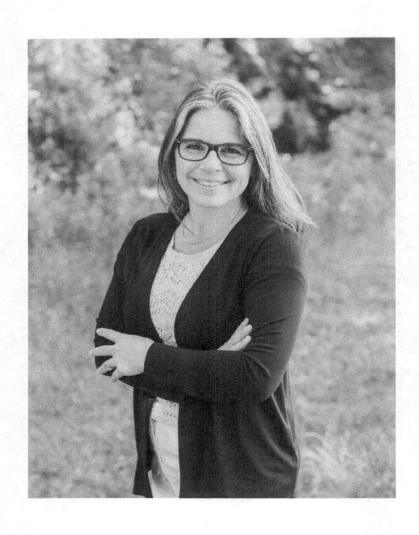

About the Author

DONNA BARTLETT, PharmD, BCGP is a Board-Certified Geriatric Pharmacist licensed in Massachusetts. She is an associate professor of pharmacy practice at the Massachusetts College of Pharmacy and Health Sciences University, with a clinical rotation site at UMASS-HealthAlliance Hospital in Leominster, MA. She has over 10 years' experience as a clinical pharmacist at the MCPHS University-Pharmacy Outreach Program, and over 20 years of retail experience. She has served as an active member of several committees, including a Pharmacy and Therapeutics Committee as a geriatric pharmacist specialist, the MA Falls Prevention Coalition, and the Poison Control and Prevention Advisory Board serving MA and RI.

She is a podcast host for *The Senior Care Pharmacist* through the American Society of Consultant Pharmacists and a guest of the *Quality Corner Show* with Pharmacy Quality Solutions. She has shared her knowledge of medication therapy management (MTM), deprescribing, polypharmacy, geriatrics, falls prevention, medication access, affordability, and adherence with various audiences, including patients, health-care providers, social workers, and professional, local, state, and national organizations. She has been published in pharmacy and managed-care journals. Donna and her husband have two children and live in Paxton, MA.

Printed in the USA
CPSIA information can be obtained
at www.ICGtesting.com
JSHW011129011023
49144JS00001B/4